SEX GAMES
BIBLE

26.04.2015.

Draga Petrice,

Želim ti svu sreću u braku sa Mirkom. Ako vam ikad ponestane

SEX GAMES BIBLE

MORE EROTIC ACTIVITIES THAN YOU COULD POSSIBLY IMAGINE TRYING

inspiracije, samo tu zavirite, sigurno

RANDI FOXX

ćete naći nešto za zanimacaju!

QUIVER

Kristina

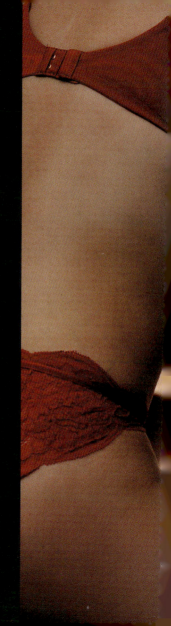

First published in the USA in 2009
by Quiver, a member of
Quarto Publishing Group USA Inc.
100 Cummings Center
Suite 406-L
Beverly, MA 01915-6101
www.quiverbooks.com

18 17 16 15 14   4 5 6 7 8

ISBN-13: 978-1-59233-393-6
ISBN-10: 1-59233-393-1

Library of Congress Cataloging-in-Publication Data
Foxx, Randi.
  Sex games bible : more erotic activities than you could
possibly imagine trying / by Randi Foxx.
      p. cm.
  Includes bibliographical references and index.
  ISBN-13: 978-1-59233-393-6
  ISBN-10: 1-59233-393-1
 1. Sex instruction. 2. Sex. 3. Sexual intercourse. 4.
Sexual excitement. 5. Adult party games. I. Title.
  HQ31.F783 2009
  306.77--dc22

                              2009001980

Printed and bound in Hong Kong

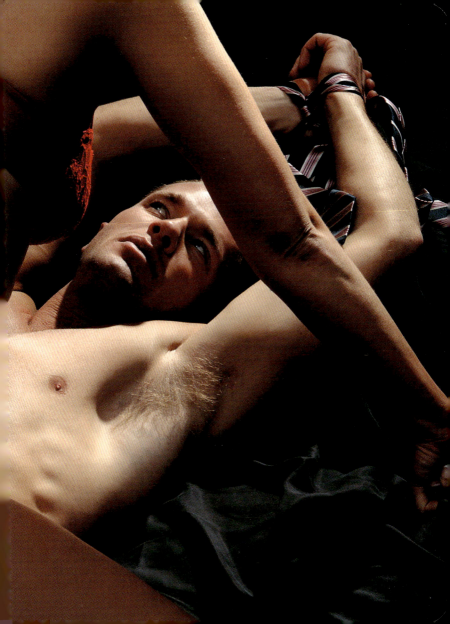

Contents

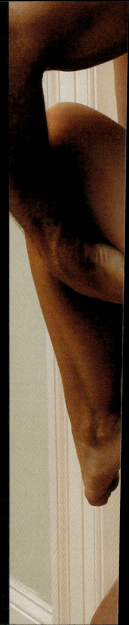

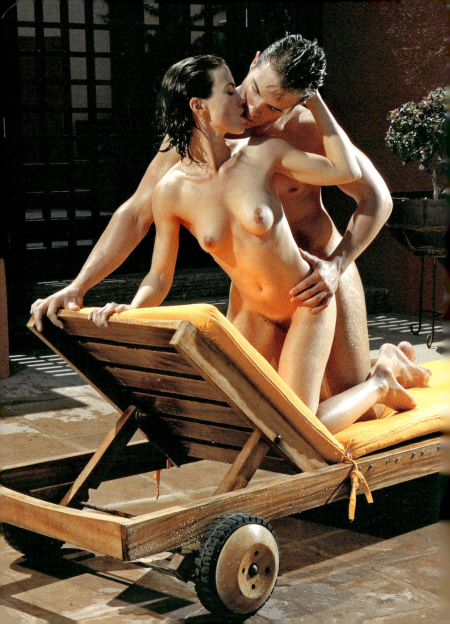

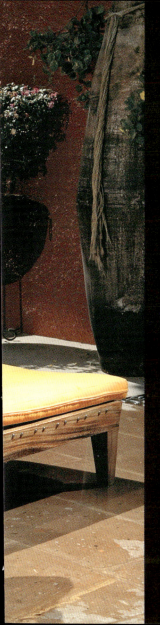

Introduction

Bored in the bedroom? Need some quick pick-me-ups for jazzing up your sex life? Then you've come to the right place. Within these pages, you'll find more fun, tantalizing, and playful games for couples, singles, and threesomes than you could ever imagine on your own.

Looking for role-playing fantasies? Look no further than chapter 6. Want to bring the sensuality of food into the bedroom? Visit chapter 2. Not sure what your sex life needs to come alive again? Flip through the book and experiment with pieces, parts, or entire games. Find a game that tickles your fancy, quickens your blood, or just brings a smile to your face, then suggest it to your lover and get ready to play. Sexual satisfaction guaranteed!

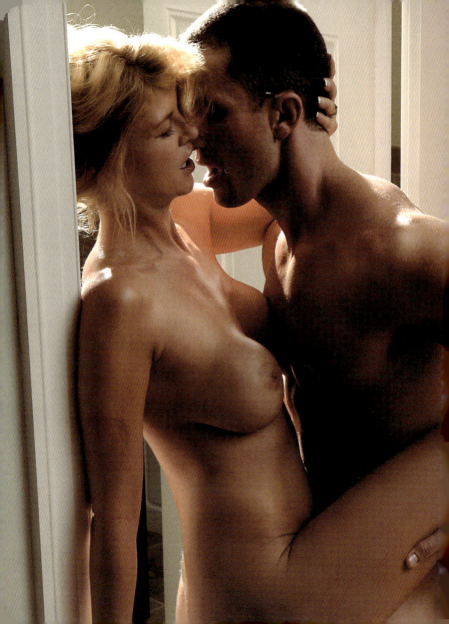

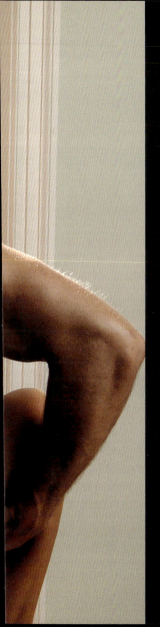

CHAPTER 1

Around the House

Think you need to leave your house to play naughty? *Au contraire!* The games in this chapter will turn every room in your house into your own personal sex playground. You'll never look at your kitchen counters or your favorite footstool the same way again.

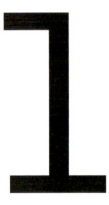

1

Soap Me Up

A hot and steamy shower is the perfect locale for this sexy, soapy game—and the hot running water will rinse away mess you might make.

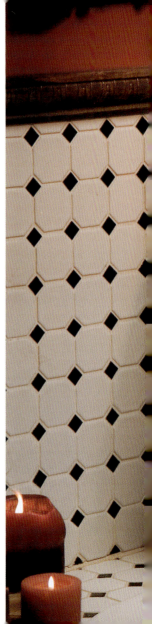

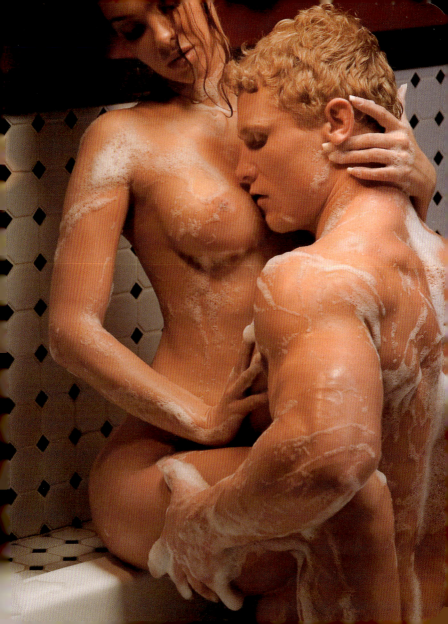

The Sexy Setup

Wake or tease your lover by kissing him on the back of the neck, then whisper that you have a soapy game in mind that's perfect for two players.

Rules & Tools

Turn the shower to nice and hot, and get the room plenty steamy to add some mystery to the scene. Get wet, lather up with your favorite soap or hand gel, and cover your breasts or genitals with bubbles.

Playing the Game

Sweet and safe: Ask your lover to stand with his face toward the shower. Soap up your hands and slowly explore every inch of your lover's backside: Caress his shoulders using a circular motion, kiss him between the shoulders, run one soapy finger down to the small of his back, use your fingernails to lightly scratch his buttocks, and suddenly (without warning) gently cup his testicles in your hands. Then finish up with a soapy hand job— from behind!

Hot and spicy: Stand facing the showerhead, and let your lover approach you from behind. Tell him to soap himself up and manhandle you, grabbing and stroking your breasts, running his soapy hands down your belly, and running a finger along your clitoris. Once he's teased you into submission, have him enter you from behind and stroke your clitoris using the bar of soap or a soapy finger.

Up the Ante

- Tell your lover your body is his for the taking, but he must use the showerhead (or the running water) to turn you on. Start by kissing together under the streaming water, letting some of the hot water catch in your mouths. Have him hold that warm water in his mouth while he kisses your breasts and nipples; for women, hold the warm water in your mouth while your suck on the head of his penis. Close your eyes and let the steam keep you warm while he uses the handheld showerhead to stimulate your clitoris.

- Add a touch of sass to the sweet and safe scenario above: Gently wash, caress, and/or explore your lover's backside and anus using a soapy hand, then rinse off the soap and move to your knees to tease and arouse him from the back using your tongue.

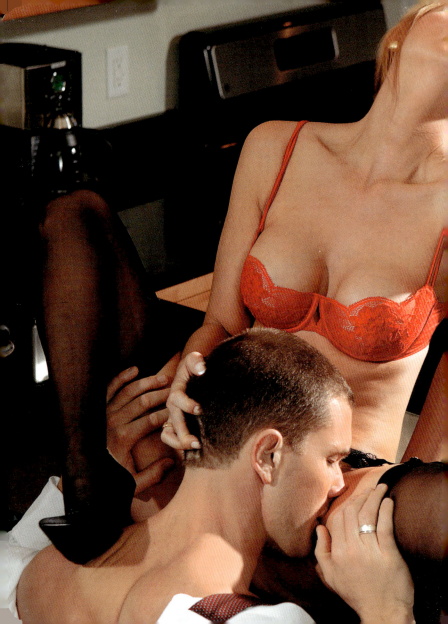

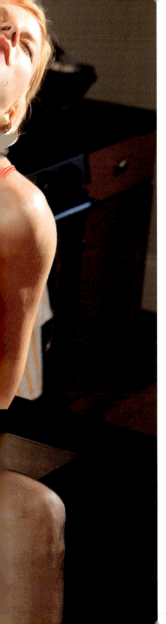

2

Preheat the Oven

Put away the pots and pans—you'll want to play this racy game of foreplay right on the kitchen counter.

The Sexy Setup

Tell your lover that your oven needs preheating. What's more, your drawers are open and you're serving something hot and spicy for dinner.

Rules & Tools

Clean off the counters and dim the lights. Wear an apron with nothing under it and line up some sexy kitchen tools or gadgets, such as a soft pastry brush or a pair of tongs (if you like it a little rougher) and don't forget the massage oil. Set the timer to however long you want the foreplay to last.

Playing the Game

Sweet and safe: Position yourself on the counter, then ask him to remove your apron using his teeth. Once you're naked, ask him to prepare you for higher temperatures by rubbing you down with massage oil. Make sure he spends ample time on your breasts, rump, and inner thighs.

Hot and spicy: Ask your lover to blindfold you with a kitchen towel and turn you on using his choice of kitchen utensils. Suggestions include tickling your inner thighs or genitals with a soft pastry brush, gently pinching you nipples with tongs, blowing cool air on your neckline using a turkey baster, and so forth.

Up the Ante

- Lie on the counter, let your lover blindfold you with a kitchen towel, and ask him to bring out a tray of ice cubes. Start by passing an ice cube back and forth between you while you kiss. Have him hold the cube in his mouth while he explores your body, alternating between an icy tongue and hot breath. The goal: Melt all the ice cubes in the tray!

- Cook together naked (except for your aprons), then feed each other by hand as foreplay.

3

Tubby Time

Remember when you were young, and tub time meant playtime? It's time to use the tub for more than just getting clean . . . and don't forget your favorite water toys.

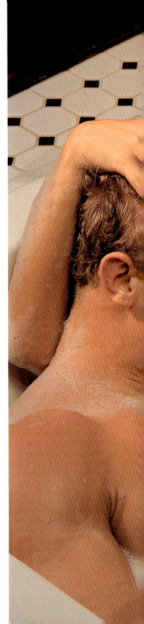

The Sexy Setup

Tell your lover you have something special planned for the bath, and you might need help reaching all your special spots. Invite her to come and play with you!

Rules & Tools

Although sex in the bath is wonderfully sensual, it can dry out your juices, so add a few drops of mineral oil to the water to keep things more lubricated. Bring along body paints (sweet and safe) or a bowl of chocolate pudding (hot and spicy). Then gather your favorite soap and tub toys, such as that vibrating rubber duck or terry mitt, and get wet!

Playing the Game

Sweet and safe: Get dirty together using body paints—paint a bull's-eye on your chest or bottom, or use arrows to mark any areas that need special attention. Paint stripes on your penis, polka dots on your testicles, and smiley faces on her breasts. Climb into the tub together and take turns washing everything off.

Hot and spicy: Use the chocolate pudding to paint yourself a G-string or her a tiny bikini, then take turns eating and licking the chocolate off. Use the pudding to play tic-tac-toe on her belly or decorate her lower back (you lick it off), or ask her to make a vanilla-chocolate mess with a gooey hand job. Put those soapsuds to work to clean it all up!

Up the Ante

- Use your tub toys creatively—put on that soft washing mitt (don't use the exfoliating version!) and have her give you a soapy hand job you'll never forget!

- Buy a sex toy that's made for the bath: The "I Rub My Duckie" vibrating rubber ducky is great for stimulating her clitoris among the bubbles!

- Ask your lover if you can shave her pubic hair, either shaping it into erotic patterns or removing it altogether.

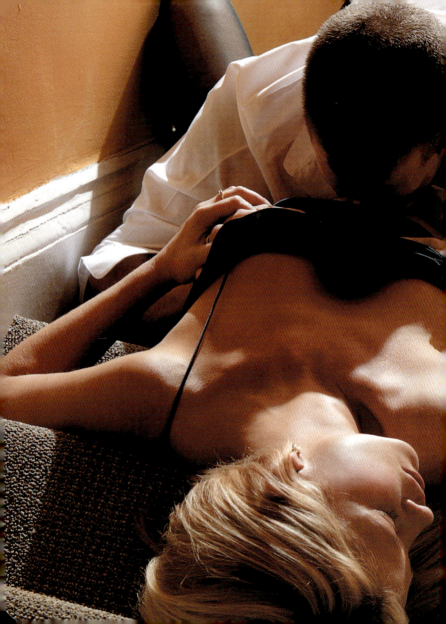

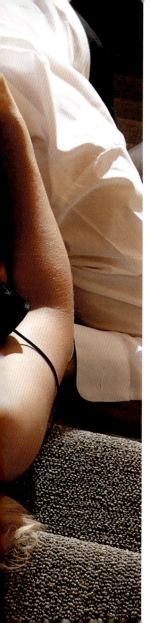

4

Stair Climber

Upstairs, downstairs—your stairs are
the perfect place for playing this game
of up and down (and in and out)!

The Sexy Setup

Leave or send your lover a suggestive note telling her to meet you on the staircase at a set time. Mention that you're dreaming of going up . . . and going down.

Rules & Tools

You should wear clothing that is easily removable: for women, a button-down shirt and zip-up skirt; for men, a button-down shirt and boxer shorts. If your stairs are not carpeted, bring out a blanket.

Playing the Game

Sweet and safe: In this version, you're (the stair "climber") in control. Have her position herself five or six stairs up, then tie one or both of her wrists to one of the banisters. Start at her toes and remove her clothing, piece by piece. You can be gentle and teasing, or get a little rough and tear or pull her clothes off. Once you come within range of her mouth, tease her by brushing your lips, belly, or penis near her face and mouth. Once she's naked, service her from your stairway position, either by spreading her legs for intercourse or having her open her mouth to suck you.

Hot and spicy: In this version, the stair climber is the slave, and you (positioned on the stairs) are the master. Position yourself three or four stairs up, completely naked, and direct your lover to start at your toes and climb, all the while licking, kissing, or exploring every inch of you. Once her face reaches your face take time to kiss passionately, but then ask her to go back down the stairs and repeat the process as needed. Your perch on the edge of the stair should give her the perfect position for exploring your manhood, but don't be afraid to grab her, position her at the edge of the stairs, and penetrate her fully.

Up the Ante

- Try either of the above games with your (or your lover's) backside facing outward.

- Blindfold the stair captive so she doesn't know what's coming next, then introduce a feather and massage oil for teasing her inner thighs, lower back, and nape of the neck.

- Move your lover to the laundry room: Have her hop on top of the washing machine or dryer and pull you into her. The vibrations will intensify every sensation!

- Pick her up and carry her, with you still inside her, to the pool table. Drive your shaft into her pocket!

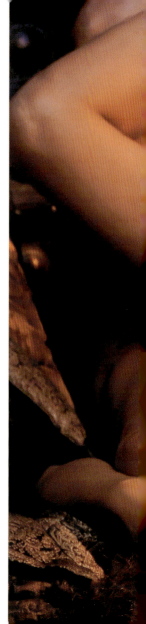

5

Fashion Show

Who doesn't like an X-rated fashion show, especially when you know it's a big turn-on for your lover?

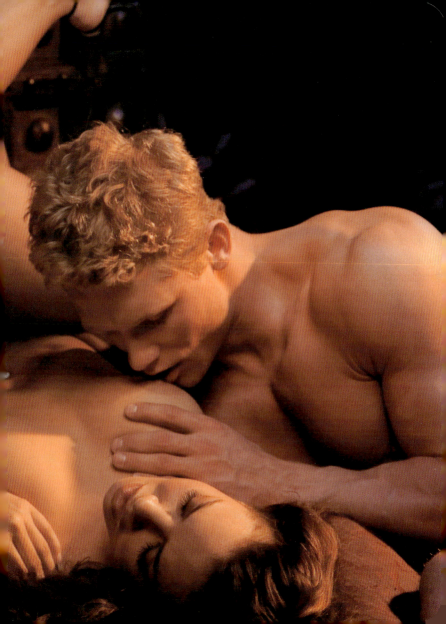

The Sexy Setup

Invite your lover to an X-rated fashion show with a suggestive note, text message, or voice mail. Mention that he can look (but not touch!) as you show off your latest line of do-me shoes and revealing outfits.

Rules & Tools

Go through your closet ahead of time and assemble four or five sexy outfits, thinking as creatively as possible. Set up a viewing chair for your partner and design your catwalk. Practice your sexy walk, teasing turns, and revealing moves in the mirror beforehand.

Playing the Game

Sweet and safe: Have a wet shirt contest and ask your partner to judge the entries. Don each shirt, jump in the shower, then strut your stuff. Experiment with light-colored T-shirts, a white button-down shirt, a sheer or satin blouse, and a skintight turtleneck. Clothing below the top is purely optional!

Hot and spicy: Don your leather jacket (with nothing underneath) and your knee- or thigh-high boots. Leather gloves, lace-up bustier, heavy chain jewelry, and fishnet stockings can add to the effect. Strut your stuff, then switch gears and contrast these shades of sadomasochism with a soft and sexy fur wrap over a sheer, see-through dress. Ask him which side of you he likes better—leather or lace? Rough or gentle? Dominant or submissive?

Up the Ante

- Sacrifice your tightest T-shirt and matching tights and cut out peekaboo holes in strategic areas. Call this the "clit and tit" ensemble and make sure he's got a front-row seat for this outfit.

- Create a bra or bikini top using silk scarves. Use a second silky scarf to create a bottom, but leave it loose so you can stimulate yourself as you strut for your lover. Capture him with a third scarf and perform a racy lap dance.

- Ask your lover to wear your sexy things for a little cross-dressing adventure!

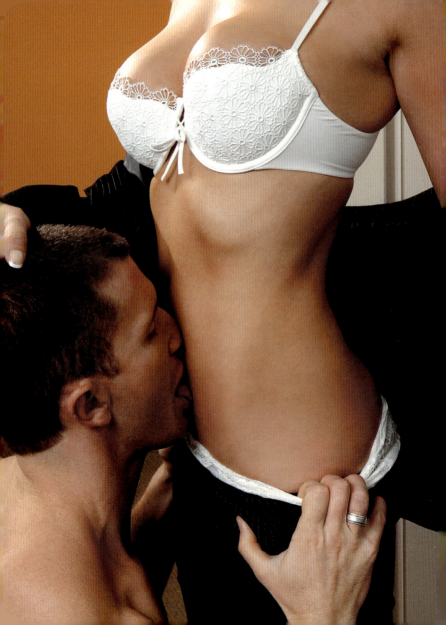

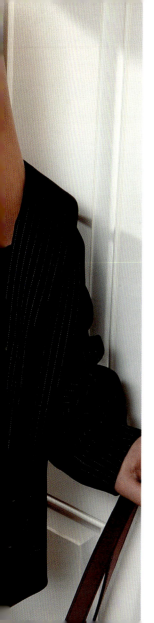

6

Strip Poker

How about a hand of cards, winner
takes all—or should we say,
winner takes *off* all?

The Sexy Setup

Play to your lover's ego and mention you'd like to play
strip poker, but you're sure *you'll* be the one doing most
of the undressing.

Rules & Tools

Set a sexy scene, take out a deck of playing cards, and
review the rules (see box). Figure out ahead of time how
the game will work: For poker, each time you lose a hand
you have to take off an article of clothing. Assemble a big
pile of coins and divide it into two sets, one for each of you.

How to play seven-card stud poker: Deal two cards
facedown and one card faceup. Make a bet (e.g., fifty
cents, one dollar, etc.), then deal three cards faceup and
the final card facedown. Winning hands (highest to lowest) are as follows: royal flush, straight flush, flush, full
house, three of a kind, two pair, one pair. One pair beats
the highest card in the hand.

Playing the Game

Sweet and safe: The winner of each hand gets to tell the other player which article of clothing to take off. See whether you can continue this drawn-out foreplay until one (or both) of you is fully undressed, then let the winner decide how he or she wants to be serviced. Consider setting satisfaction rules, such as only using your hands or your mouth.

Hot and spicy: The winner of each hand gets to command the loser to take off an article of clothing and perform a service, such as "massage my feet," "stroke my breasts," or "suck on the tip of my penis." Continue this drawn-out card play/foreplay until one of you is fully undressed. At this point, switch over to a fantasy game where your lover becomes a card shark and you're a gambler who has run out of money (or vice versa). The card shark gets to decide how you will pay off your debt, whether that means sucking him off or performing other services to his satisfaction.

Up the Ante

- Invite friends over for a group game of strip poker. Set some ground rules beforehand (unless you don't mind hosting a game of swap partners or swinging 101!).

7

Strip
Scrabble

How about a game of Strip Scrabble,
where you can watch your lover undress
and win points for spelling dirty words?

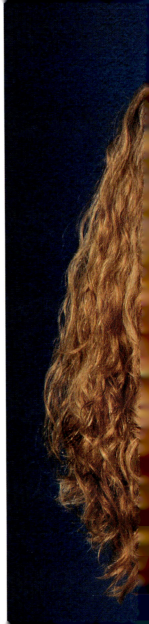

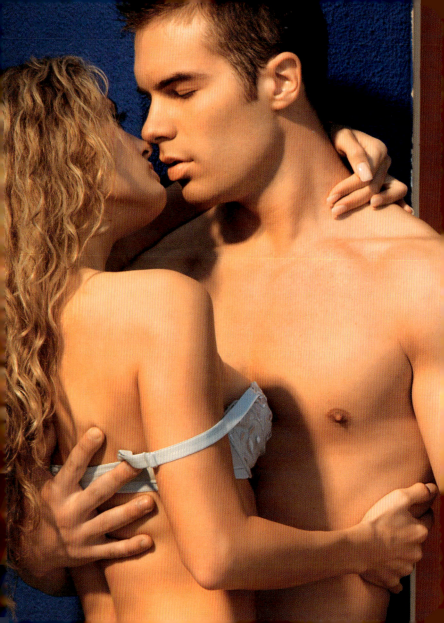

The Sexy Setup

Tell your lover you have a board game that certainly won't be boring. Tell her to get ready for some wordplay that might lead to foreplay.

Rules & Tools

You'll need a Scrabble board game. Set a sexy scene by turning down the lights, lighting a few candles, and pouring some wine.

Playing the Game

Sweet and safe: Play Scrabble, but for each round the player with the lower scoring word must take off a piece of clothing. Continue playing until you're both naked (and let nature takes its course!) or until one player wins. The winner gets to pick the position, fantasy, or location for your sexy exploration.

Hot and spicy: Spell out dirty or sexy words or phrases, such as *kissme* or *lickhere*. Add in the strip factor if desired, or require the player with the lower scoring word to demonstrate his or her word or phrase.

Up the Ante

- Make up new words or phrases to describe sexy maneuvers. With each round, award extra "sexual favor" points for creativity, or make the player with the lowest scoring word or phrase demonstrate the maneuver.

- Turn your other favorite board games into "sex" games: Backgammon, Uno, even "War" with a deck of cards can be dirty!

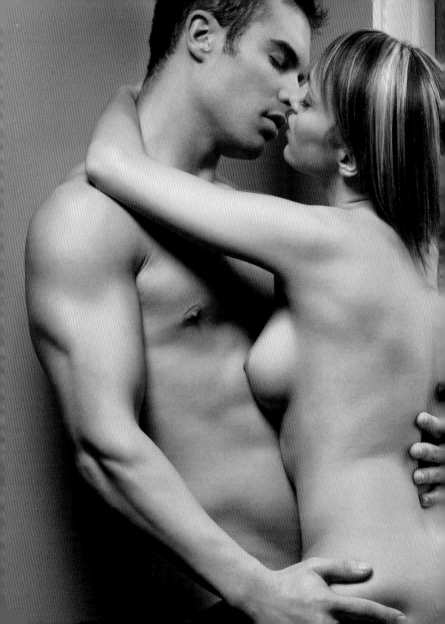

8

Strip Monopoly

How about a game of Strip Monopoly,
with sex on the boardwalk
a most definite option?

The Sexy Setup

Invite your lover to a special game night, but tell her to be ready for more than just buying properties, riding the railroad, or passing GO!

Rules & Tools

You'll need a Monopoly board game. Choose a sexy location and dim the lights, light some candles, and assemble some pillows and blankets on the floor.

Playing the Game

Sweet and safe: Play the game, but set up rules for stripping, such as remove one article of clothing each time you roll doubles, pass "GO," or visit Community Chest. Continue playing until you're both undressed, one player wins, or something in between!

Hot and spicy: When you land on another player's property, assign other "duties" that must be performed in addition to paying rent, such as a quick French kiss or a gentle grope of the breast. Be creative and make up new rules: Anyone who gets sent to jail has to perform a sexual act on the other player, or anyone who lands on Community Chest has to flash the other player.

Up the Ante

- Add some new rules to your dice play: Anyone who rolls double 1s, for example, gets a quick massage; double 2s a french kiss, and so on . . .

- Count up the money at the end of the game and determine how much money the winner won by. Then "spend" your money in a role-playing game of Hooker and Customer. (The player with the most amount of money gets to decide who gets serviced and who does the servicing.) Assign fees for services: $500 for a blow job, $350 for a hand job, $200 for straight intercourse, and so on!

9

Naughty Nap Time

Here's a naughty game that's purrrrrfect for a lazy Sunday afternoon at home.

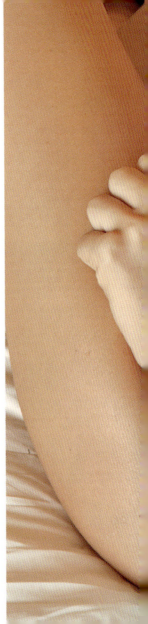

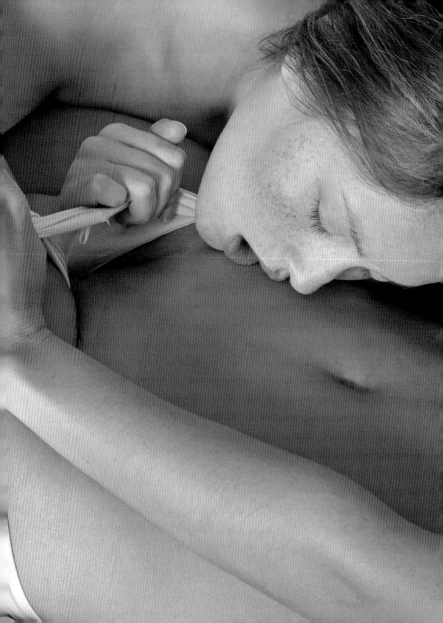

The Sexy Setup

Write your lover a naughty note, spray it with a new fragrance or cologne, and leave it by his coffee or put it in his coat pocket. Write something like this: "Breathe in the scent of this note. Each time you smell this scent on me in the coming days you will have an uncontrollable desire to go into the bedroom and take a nap. Once you lie down, you are not allowed to open your eyes, speak, or use your hands, no matter what happens."

Rules & Tools

You can stick with your favorite scent of perfume or cologne (sweet and safe) or body lotion (hot and spicy) or, better yet, buy something new for the occasion— the sexier the better!

Playing the Game

Sweet and safe: Spray on your new scent and cuddle up to your lover. Ask him if he likes the smell, then remind him of your note. Give him a few minutes to get to the bedroom, then quietly enter the room. Be as quiet as possible as you blindfold and then undress your lover.

Kiss him all over; as your man gets excited, gently touch the area between his scrotum and anus, making him squirm for more. When the time is right, climb on top of him and bring him to orgasm.

Hot and spicy: Write the same type of note, but in addition to spraying it with perfume or cologne, also attach a small amount of lotion in a small plastic bag. Once your lover gets to the bedroom, warm up the lotion in your hands, then give him a sensual massage with plenty of teasing moves and loving caresses. When the time is right, lube up your hand (or fingers) and bring your lover to a wet and creamy orgasm.

Up the Ante

- Sign the note "Your Venus Butterfly." Then teach him how to perform this much talked about sexual technique: He should use his tongue on your clitoris, place several fingers in your vagina and use the other hand to stroke your buttocks or penetrate your anus. Be prepared for a multifaceted orgasm! (Women can perform a variation of this by sucking on his penis, cupping his testicles or stroking behind his balls with one hand, and slipping a finger into his anus with the other hand.)

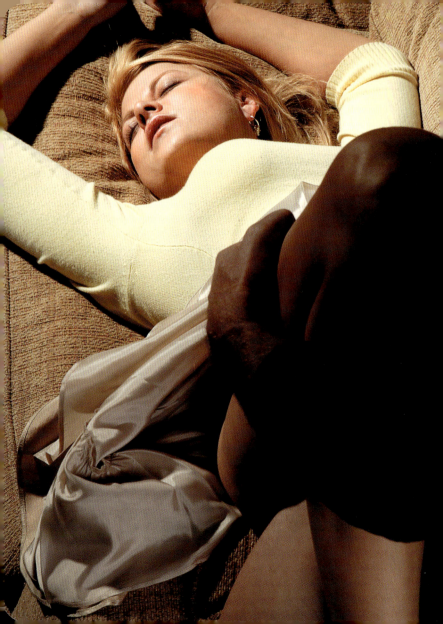

10

Movie Night

What's your favorite sexy movie?
It's time to rent it, then reinvent it!
This game revolves around the
sexy food scene in *9½ Weeks* staring
Mickey Rourke and Kim Basinger,
but you can alter it to fit any of
your favorite sexy scenes.

The Sexy Setup

Buy a blonde wig, fishnet stockings, and a sexy bra. Take a photo of yourself with your face covered and send it to your lover with a message that Kim Basinger (or the actress of your choice) wants him to come over and play.

Rules & Tools

Rent the movie beforehand (if necessary) and study the food and/or sex scenes. Assemble an assortment of sensual foods, such as strawberries, pineapple, olives, and the like.

Playing the Game

Sweet and safe: Watch the movie together, wearing your blonde wig, fishnet stockings, and sexy bra. Take special note of the food scene, then tell him you'd like to reenact it. Take turns being the seducer (Mickey Rourke) and the seduced (Kim Basinger).

Hot and spicy: Reenact the movie scene, but make your own video at the same time. Pick out an assortment of racy scenes (from this film or others) and let the cameras roll!

Up the Ante

- Create an entire library of sexy reenactments. Consider *Striptease* (starring Demi Moore), *Exotica* (starring Mia Kirshner), or *Fatal Attraction* (starring Michael Douglas and Glenn Close).

OTHER SEXY MOVIES

Need more ideas? Try renting these notoriously racy films:

Secretary (starring Maggie Gyllenhaal)

Two Moon Junction (starring Sherilyn Fenn)

Bound (starring Jennifer Tilly)

Unfaithful (starring Diane Lane)

Lie with Me (starring Lauren Lee Smith)

Lake Consequences (starring Billy Zane)

Bolero (starring Bo Derek)

Wild Things (starring Matt Dillon)

Lolita (starring Jeremy Irons)

Sex, Lies, and Videotape (starring James Spader)

Risky Business (starring Tom Cruise)

The Lover (starring Jane March)

White Palace (starring Susan Sarandon)

Betty Blue (starring Jean-Hugues Anglade)

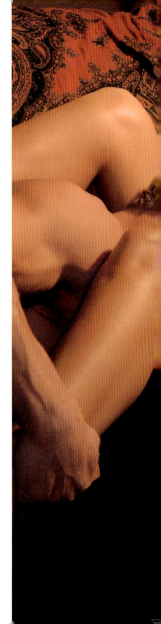

11

Blue Velvet

Nothing to do on a Saturday night?
Play this sweet and naughty game
of pain-and-pleasure using your
softest fabrics.

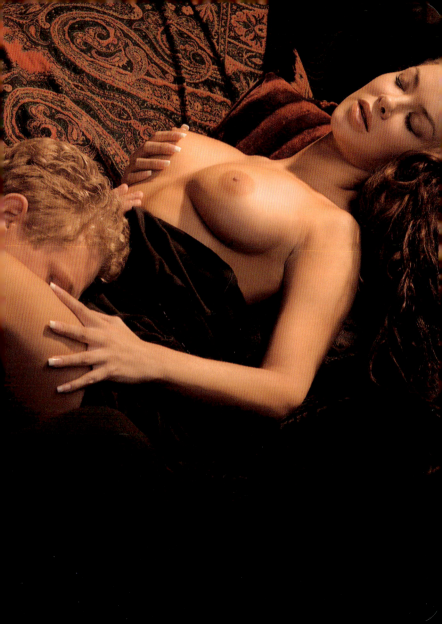

The Sexy Setup

Send your lover a note telling him about the special room
in your house devoted to pleasure. In it, there's a bed of
velvet and fake fur blankets. Your lover is invited to spend
a few hours in this sensual heaven, with you as the mistress
of erotic pleasure.

Rules & Tools

Assemble your softest, most sensual fabrics and focus on
making your bed (or couch) a zone of pleasure for the skin.
Make a quick trip to the fabric store and buy some velvet
or velour castoffs to create a soft, velvety area for your
lover to lie on, then pull out your softest cashmere sweater
or wrap, silk scarves or gloves, fur accessories, a feather,
and any other clothing or fabric that feels good on bare
skin. When your lover arrives, blindfold him and lead him
into the pleasure chamber. For the hot and spicy version
of the game, be sure to have some ice cubes or a popsicle
on hand.

Playing the Game

Sweet and safe: Use the various fabrics to touch his entire body. Slowly sweep the silk across his nipples, tease his inner thighs with a caress of velvet, and tickle his lower back with a brush of fur. Massage and caress your lover with each fabric, but avoid the genitals on purpose. Occasionally brush your nipples across his face, or lightly kiss his lower back. Eventually your travels lead you to massaging his penis with velvet-, fur-, or cashmere-covered hands.

Hot and spicy: Use one fabric at a time to stroke his penis and ask him to guess what each one is. If he gets it wrong, run an ice cube or Popsicle over his nipples, penis, or testicles for an exciting, icy jolt (make it quick, otherwise it might be painful. On the other hand, some lovers like mixing pain with pleasure . . .). If he guesses correctly, reward him with a deep, passionate kiss.

Up the Ante

- Tie your lover's hands together using a length of velvet or silk, then tease his neck, chest, nipples, belly, inner thighs, lower back, penis, or testicles with the other fabrics. Try to bring your lover to orgasm using just the touch of fabric—silk on the clitoris, and so on.

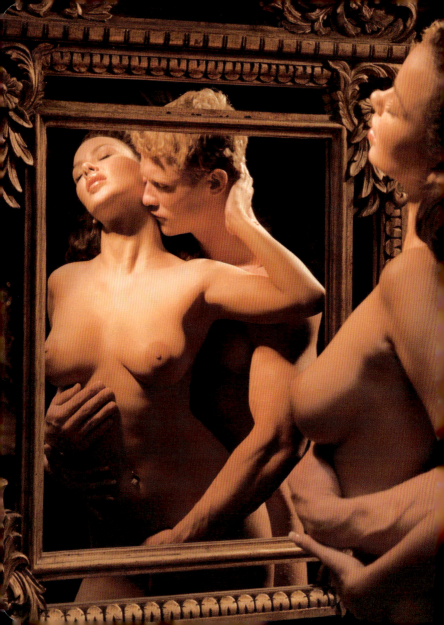

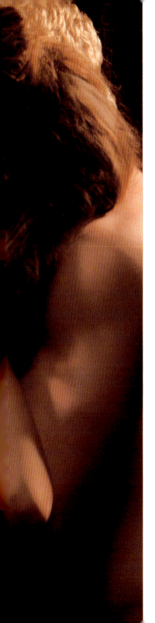

12

Anatomy
Lessons

Time for a series of close-up and personal
anatomy lessons with you as the teacher
and your lover as the model.

The Sexy Setup

Tell your lover that you are the teacher, she's the model, and today's lesson is anatomy. She's expected to sit, listen, and learn without moving or touching her personal instructor.

Rules & Tools

You'll need a handheld mirror. Have her dress in a short, sexy robe. For the art class model game, you'll need a pencil and sketchpad, a chair or stool, and an artist's paintbrush.

Playing the Game

Sweet and safe: Ask her to hold the mirror while you gently teach her the basics of anatomy, starting at the neck and moving downward. Examine and discuss her various assets in detail. Next, demonstrate what happens when you touch, stroke, or fondle her breasts, nipples, and other body parts (or try handling them more aggressively!). She has to watch, holding the handheld mirror, while you demonstrate just what happens when the touching continues (and the talking stops!).

Hot and spicy: Once the basic lesson is complete, you hold the mirror so she can demonstrate what happens when the instructor leaves the room. (She should masturbate while you hold the mirror.) Then swap roles, and let her be the instructor while you serve as the model.

Up the Ante

- Pretend she's a nude model for an art class, and ask her to pose naked while you sketch her. As an art student, you can ask her to assume certain poses or positions; as a model, she must do whatever you say. Once you're done with the sketch, use an artist's paintbrush to tease her body, including brushing gently between the buttocks, along the inner thighs, and all around the ''v'' of her genitals.

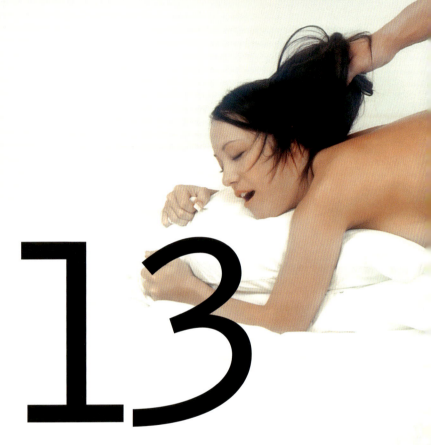

13

Pillow Pleasures

Fluff up the pillows! This game of domination uses pillows to prop up your lover for deep penetration or hands-on action.

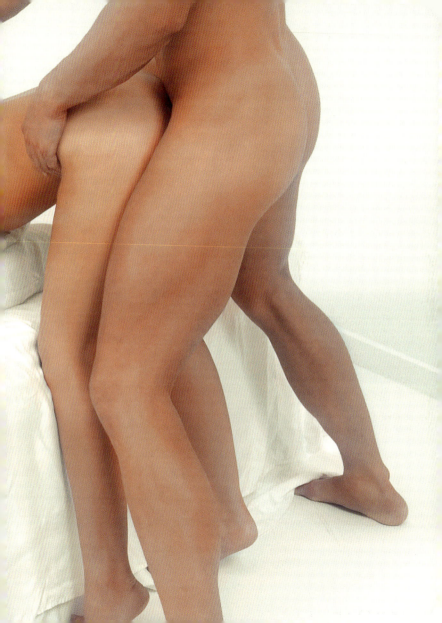

The Sexy Setup

Guys, tell your lover you're the boss, and you have a game that's just right for proving your manhood.

Rules & Tools

Gather some pillows for propping up your lover and to give you a commanding view of the situation.

Playing the Game

Sweet and safe: Have her stand in front of you, then lean over onto a bed or couch, lifting her backside into the air. You command the situation, whether you want to see her touch herself or just get down to action and pull her hair, manhandle her breasts, or penetrate her deeply from behind. Tease her by pushing in and pulling out slowly— your commanding view of the penetration should turn you on!

Hot and spicy: This time she's in command. Bend over onto the pillows, exposing your backside for pleasure (or pain). She can tease your testicles with her tongue and nip at your buttocks with her teeth, pull your hair, or man-handle your penis, all the while commanding you to fulfill her every wish. If she enjoys the position of power, let her tease you until you're begging for release, then flip over so she can jump on top and ride you straight to heaven!

Up the Ante

- Add some spanking to either scenario, along with a few gentle slaps, to make your pillow play a little rougher.

- Have a pillow fight in the nude!

- Have her lay on her back and prop up her genitals using a pillow. Lavish attention on her "mound" until you bring her to orgasm!

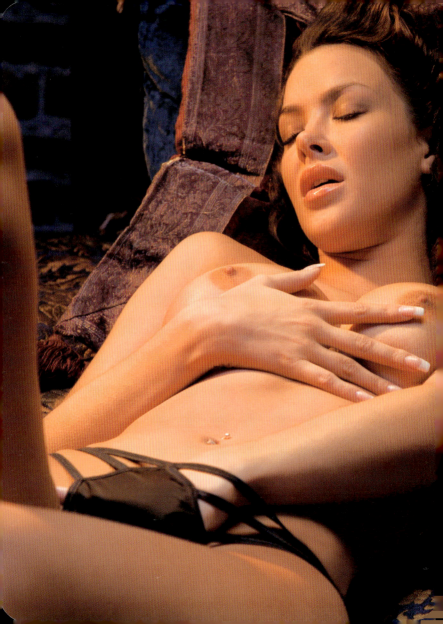

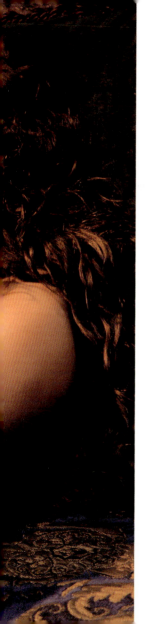

14

Show and Tell

Here's a game of voyeurism and exhibition:
Make your lover his own personal video
of you pleasuring yourself . . .
with him as the narrator.

The Sexy Setup

Ask your lover if he likes to imagine you touching yourself, then tell him you're going to give him a personal demonstration that he can watch over and over again.

Rules & Tools

You'll need a video camera and stand. Scout out several sexy locations, such as a bathtub full of bubbles, a doorway and a silk scarf, or a bed of velvet or fake furs.

Playing the Game

Sweet and safe: Set up the camera after you've filled the tub (this keeps the steam from fogging up the lens). Add a candle and scatter some fresh-cut roses in and around the tub. Get in and soap yourself slowly and enticingly. Have enough bubble coverage to invoke a little mystery and work your way from innocently washing yourself to pleasuring yourself, complete with moans and cries of pleasure.

Hot and spicy: Set up the camera, then stand in front of your closet, pretending you're trying to find something to wear. Strip slowly out of your clothing, taking extra time in front of the camera as you slip out of your undergarments or remove your bra, fondling your own breasts as you slide off your clothing. Open the closet, pull out a silk scarf, and drape it around your neck, letting the silky ends tickle your buttocks or breasts. Lift one leg up onto a dressing stool or an open dresser drawer and run the scarf across your genital region. (Make sure the camera is directed toward your breasts and genitals). Close your eyes, continue stroking yourself with the scarf, and finally bring yourself to orgasm, cooing and moaning to add sound effects.

Up the Ante

- Tell your lover you'd like to make a film of him pleasuring himself. Set him up in the bathtub or on a bed of furs, then ask him to turn himself on and bring himself to orgasm while you film. Be prepared to drop the camera and join the action if you can't hold back!

- Play film school, with the person behind the camera learning how to produce and direct, and you the budding star. Remember, the producer gets to pose the starlet (or vice versa) in any pose he or she likes!

15

Talk It Up

Imagine teasing your lover to death
using just words, and you have the
gist of this game that's perfect
for any room in the house.

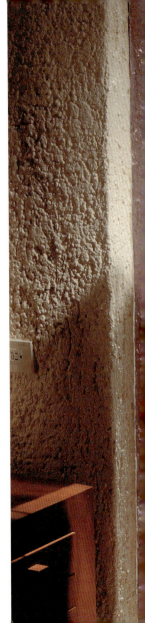

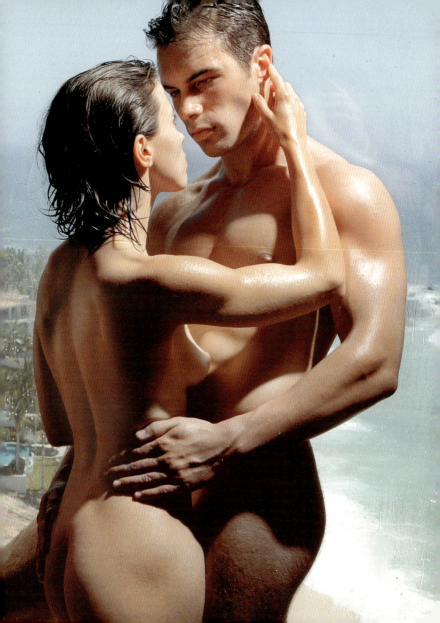

The Sexy Setup

Tell your lover you have a teasing game that's sure to turn her on and it only involves one tool: your voices.

Rules & Tools

Turn off all the lights and sit in a room together, completely naked. Remember, no touching allowed! The goal is to tease and turn each other on just by talking, whispering suggestively, or issuing commands.

Playing the Game

Sweet and safe: Take turns describing all the nasty, naughty things you want to do to your lover. After that, ask questions like "What part of my body turns you on the most?" or "Which do you prefer, my sucking on your nipples or your clitoris?"

Tell her how sexy she is, and describe how you love touching the various parts of her body. Be as graphic and as detailed as you feel comfortable. As you start getting excited, tell your lover you're going to pleasure yourself, then explain, in graphic detail, what you're doing, how it feels, and how you like to be touched.

Hot and spicy: Talk dirty or ask her to play hooker/slut. If she's playing hooker, have her describe what she gets paid for (sucking big dicks, etc.). Have her tell you why she's the right hooker for you, and what she will do to turn you on.

Up the Ante

- Use the darkness to describe your wildest fantasy. Here's one example: "I've always imagined a rough love/rape fantasy where I pull you into a darkened room, tear off your clothing, kiss you deeply all over, and penetrate you while you try to fight me off. Does that turn you on?" (If so, continue.)

- Decorate yourself with glow-in-the-dark body paint before you get undressed. Imagine her surprise when the lights go out but your genitals are on display!

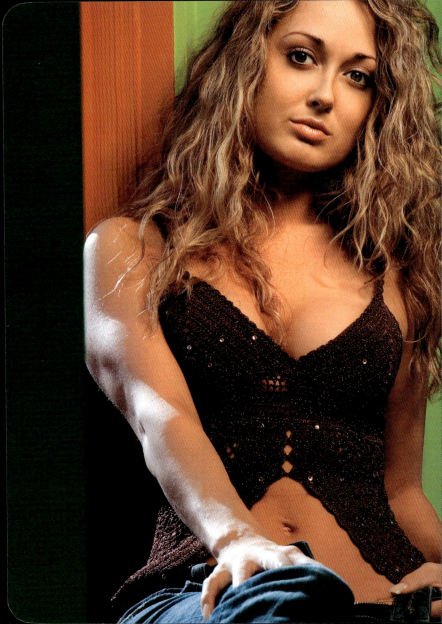

16

Striptease

Who doesn't love the idea of a striptease, performed by candlelight for a soft and sexy show, or under the pulsating vibrations of a strobe light for a more erotic version?

The Sexy Setup

Tell your lover he's invited to his own private strip club—
and his private dancer will perform any move he desires.

Rules & Tools

Purchase candles (for a romantic setting) or a strobe light
(available at party stores) for a more erotic setting. Set
up some background music to fit the role you're going to
play: soft and sexy for a one-on-one strip routine; pulsating, harder rock for the strobe light show; or exotic, seductive music for some belly dancing. Remember this key to
a good striptease: Keep your eyes locked on your partner
while removing your clothing or making your moves.

Playing the Game

Sweet and safe: Light as many candles as possible, and
dress in clothing that can be easily removed, such as a
dress or blouse that buttons down the front or a skirt that
zips at the side. Don't forget the sexy lingerie underneath!
Remove your clothing piece by piece, taking time to push
up your breasts, lean over seductively, and tease him by
coming close, then moving away.

Hot and spicy: Get the room completely dark, and wear clothes that you can easily tear off. Turn on the strobe light and perform a striptease—the light will turn your maneuvers into a series of erotic snapshots with one sexually charged image after another.

Up the Ante

- Put on some Middle Eastern music, darken under your eyes with makeup, wrap yourself in scarves and chunky jewelry, and gyrate like an exotic belly dancer. Dip and sway to the music, and remove your scarves slowly and seductively, all the while arching your back, running your hand over your nipples or belly, and swaying your hips invitingly.

- Hire a stripper or an exotic dancer to visit you and your lover at home, and be sure to tell him (or her) that you're both the guests of honor. Or visit an upscale strip club together and get a private dance to enjoy as a couple.

17

"Horny on Line One"

This is a great game for those nights when your lover is traveling on business or you're off on a girl's weekend at the spa.

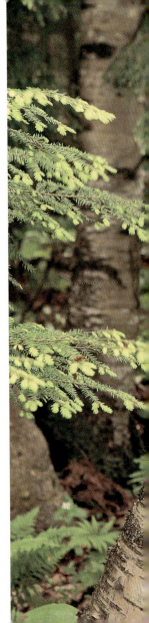

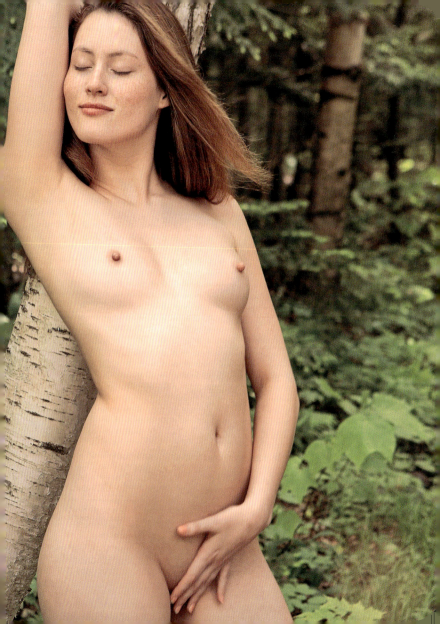

The Sexy Setup

Tell your lover you need him to set aside some private time on the phone with you tonight—clothing optional, of course. Alternatively, get his juices flowing by leaving an erotic voice mail, email, or text message.

Rules & Tools

If you need to, practice your sultry, sexy voice beforehand. You might also want to learn some new erotic lingo for describing his body parts and yours. Before you dial, dim the lights, sip some wine, or look at some erotic pictures to get your juices flowing. Tell your lover anything goes, including pleasuring himself while you talk. Have your vibrator on hand, too.

Playing the Game

Sweet and safe: First time having phone sex? Try an opening line like "I wish you were lying here with me." Then proceed to tell him what you're wearing, how it feels to slip off each piece of clothing, or how your erect nipples feel to your own fingers. The goal is to paint him a picture that's alluring and erotic.

Ask him questions, such as "Do you want to kiss my nipples?" or "Do you want to feel how wet I'm getting?" Start touching yourself, and describe every effect and sensation—your erect nipples, your soft skin, your tingling clitoris. Bring yourself to orgasm, and don't forget the sound effects: Soft moans, sighs of pleasure, throaty groans, or heavy breathing can add to the pleasure!

Hot and spicy: Tell him to get naked and begin stroking himself. As he touches himself, tell him you're imagining what his penis feels like, how hard and large he is, and what an incredibly sexy man he is. As he begins to get turned on, describe what you'd be doing if you were there—kissing his chest, licking his shaft, rubbing his buttocks, or sucking his testicles. As he brings himself to orgasm, urge him on and tell him how hot he's making you. Then turn up your vibrator and let him listen in on the action while you get off!

Up the Ante

- Ask your lover how he would feel if you tied his hands together, if you and a friend ganged up on him together, or if he'd like you to try something different, like anal penetration. Then go on to describe the situation that turns him on the most.

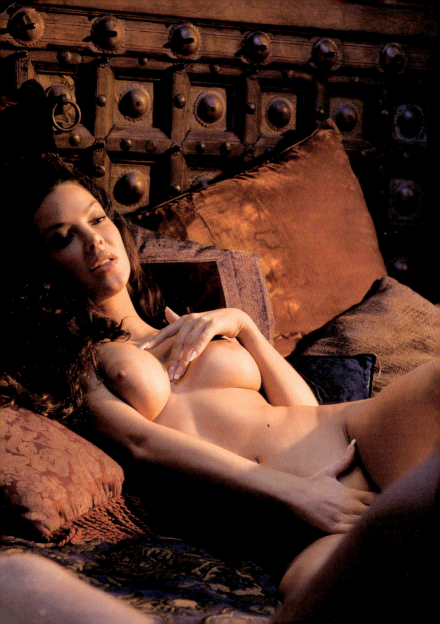

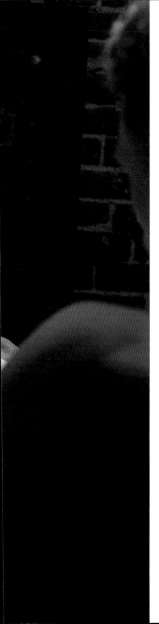

18

Pretty in Pearls

This game of making pearl jewelry using your ejaculation proves that intercourse doesn't require a mouth or vagina.

The Sexy Setup

Tell your lover you bought her a new piece of jewelry:
a pearl necklace. Mention that you also picked up a
matching pearl belt, a pearl pendant, and a lapful
of pearls in case she's interested.

Rules & Tools

There's one rule to this game: you have to get off using
any part of her body *except* an orifice. Set a sexy scene,
and create a love nest of blankets for your encounter.
Dim the lights, put on some soft music, and begin kissing
her deeply.

Playing the Game

Sweet and safe: Tell your lover you want to give her a
pearl necklace. To do this, have her lie down, then kneel
over her body, facing her, and press her breasts around
your penis. Thrust back and forth in the space created
by her breasts, adding massage oil or lubrication if it's
needed. When you're ready to come, direct your ejaculation toward her throat, thus creating droplets of semen
on her neck (a.k.a. a pearl necklace).

Hot and spicy: Ask your lover if you can give her a matching pearl belt by making love to her buttocks. Hold her cheeks around your penis, again adding massage oil or lubrication if needed, and thrust away. When you come, you'll add droplets of semen on her lower back (a.k.a. a pearl belt).

Up the Ante

- Create a fountain of pearls in her lap by having her sit on your lap and close her thighs around your penis. Add massage oil if needed.

- Give her a pearl pendant by inserting your penis between her arm and her body, or the space of her armpit. Direct your ejaculation toward the center of her chest to create this one-of-a-kind piece of jewelry!

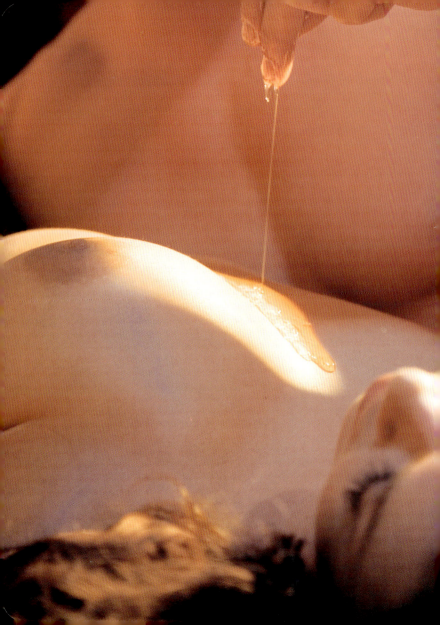

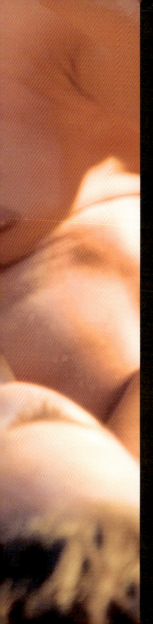

CHAPTER 2

Fun with Food

Think food is just for eating? Think again! Tempting your lover with strawberries, drizzling honey on your lover's breasts, and using fruits and vegetables for play-time are just the beginning!

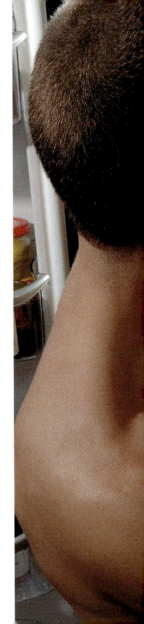

19

Make Me Your Own Sundae

Dessert's on me—literally! Let your lover build his own sundae using you as the dish.

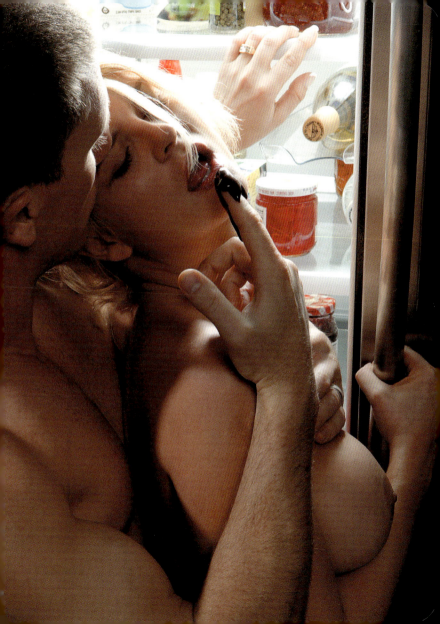

The Sexy Setup

Mention there's something special in the works for dessert, and he better get home before everything melts. The menu includes mountains of luscious whipped cream, gooey chocolate syrup, creamy caramel sauce, sweetened maraschino cherries, firm, peeled bananas—and, of course, *you*!

Rules & Tools

Have all of the "menu" items ready and just before your lover comes into the room, sit naked on the counter, dip a finger into the chocolate, and spread your legs seductively.

Playing the Game

Sweet and safe: Hand feed him cherries, let him lick chocolate off your fingers, and smear whipped cream on your belly. Then ask him to follow the trail of caramel leading downward with his tongue . . .

Hot and spicy: Dip your nipples in melted chocolate, outline your breasts in whipped cream, smear caramel on your inner thighs, and put a cherry in your belly button. Use this command: *Devour me!*

Up the Ante

- Hide the cherry between your legs and ask your lover to find it.

- Cover your clitoris with whipped cream and have him lick it off.

- Masturbate with the banana (while he watches) and have him eat the remains.

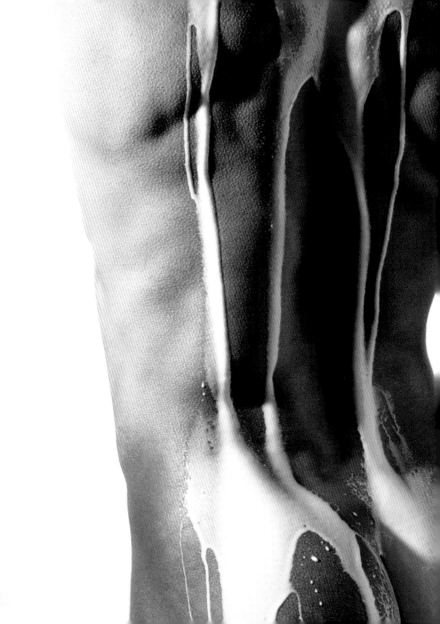

20

Milky Spa Bath

Try this sexy game in the tub, where you
give your lover a milky spa massage and
get ready to lick her all over.

The Sexy Setup

Tell your lover it's time to play spa, and you're the sexy spa attendant who's going to give her a tongue bath. Ask her to get into something comfortable, like a short robe, and get ready for a sensuous bathtub massage right at home.

Rules & Tools

Make the bathroom mysterious and romantic by dimming the lights and lighting some candles; putting out some clean, fluffy towels; and assembling a bath pillow, soft wash mitt, body wash, and a bottle or jar of milk-based moisturizer (to stick with the theme). Buy two or three gallons of milk and use a large pot on the stove to heat it up; make sure it's not too hot! Fill the tub about halfway with hot water.

Playing the Game

Sweet and safe: Ask your lover to climb into the tub and get comfortable. Transfer the milk to a pitcher or pouring device, then slowly pour some of the milk onto your lover's head, neck, chest, and arms.

Start from the fingertips and lick every inch of your partner's body, leaving not a single patch of milk-covered skin untouched. Continue pouring and licking, or add in a milky massage, a sensuous shampoo, or an all-over body wash.

Hot and spicy: Pour the milk onto your lover's breasts and nipples, then suck her nipples like a baby and lick her clean like a cat. Use the milk to lubricate your hands, then massage and tease her belly and thighs. Have her lean back on the bath pillow, then ask her to spread her legs. Pour milk onto her genitals, then stimulate her clitoris using your fingers. Bring her to orgasm using lubrication or a waterproof vibrator.

Up the Ante

- Continue the spa experience once you're done washing your lover. Help her out of the tub and rub her dry with clean towels, then ask her to lie down while you moisturize and massage her entire body using the milk-based moisturizer. Don't let her do the touching—this is all about giving her pleasure!

Chocolate Syrup Scavenger Hunt

Who doesn't love a scavenger hunt? This naughty version involves hunting for hidden pockets of chocolate syrup delight.

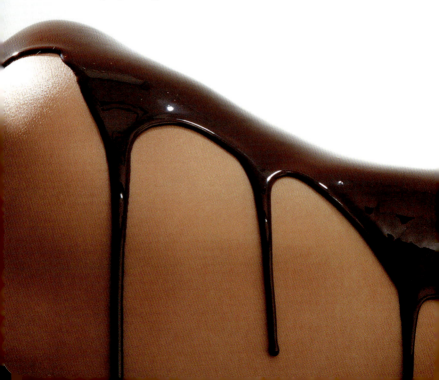

21

The Sexy Setup

Tell your lover it's time for a scavenger hunt, but this time she is searching for tiny drops or puddles of chocolate syrup—on your naked body.

Rules & Tools

You'll need a blindfold and chocolate syrup. Consider playing this game on a sheet or blanket that can be easily washed.

Playing the Game

Sweet and safe: Blindfold your lover and have her stay close by. Choose three places on your body to pour a few drops or a nickel-size puddle of chocolate syrup, then tell her she must find the sweet treasure using only her tongue. No peeking!

Hot and spicy: Let her be the artist! Ask her to blindfold you, decorate your body with chocolate syrup, and lick it all off. Suggest she dribble syrup into your navel, use her fingers to smear chocolate on your inner thighs, or encircle your nipples. You won't know where the chocolate's going, or which direction your lover's tongue will be traveling.

Up the Ante

- Invite your lover to eat his favorite dessert: clitoral chocolate delight. Dribble chocolate syrup on or around your clitoris, spoon whipped cream onto your labia, and top it all with tiny sprinkles. Yum, yum!

- Decorate his backside with chocolate syrup, whipped cream, and sprinkles, then eat it all off while licking from his anus all the way around to the tip of his penis!

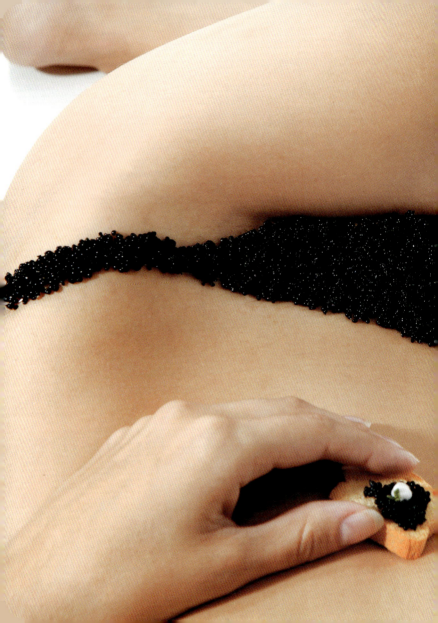

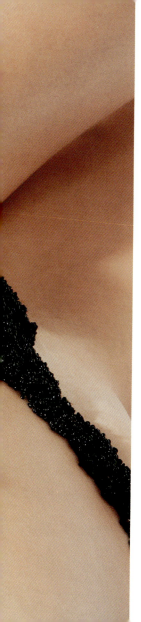

22

Picnic by Candlelight

Try this feast for the senses right in the comfort and privacy of your living room . . . just be sure to draw the shades!

The Sexy Setup

Send your lover a note and invite him to a sumptuous candlelight picnic just for the two of you. Tell him the menu includes a taste of all his favorite finger foods, such as chocolate, olives, and other tasty tidbits. Mention the dress is very casual: He should wear his finest silk boxers for this private meal.

Rules & Tools

Light a fire in the fireplace, or, if you don't have a fireplace, fill your living room with candles. (Even if you do have a fireplace, candles will heighten the mood.) Prepare some of your favorite finger foods and spread a blanket on the floor, but make sure it's one that you don't mind getting a little messy.

Playing the Game

Sweet and safe: Dress yourself in a sexy nightgown and ask him to wear silk boxers. Open your favorite champagne or wine. Lay out an extravagant feast that you can eat with your fingers, like chocolate kisses, olives, or melon wrapped in prosciutto.

For a special treat, serve caviar on a bed of crushed ice, with a small spoon to ladle it onto pieces of toast. Serve decadent chocolate truffles or juicy berries dipped in whipped cream for dessert. Feed each other the foods, and be sure to savor every bite before moving on to the next. If you spill anything, lick up your mess.

Hot and spicy: After you've had enough of tasting the food, taste each other. Disrobe each other slowly. Slide your tongue over your lover's skin. Taste his lips, his neck, and his nipples. When you kiss, prolong the exploration of each other's mouths. Relish the taste and aroma of all his body parts. Have your lover fill his mouth with champagne and trickle the bubbles over your nipples or clitoris; before you perform fellatio, take a sip of bubbly and wrap your mouth around his penis for an amazing sensation.

Up the Ante

- Use the finger foods to stimulate and tease your partner. Rub a tiny pickle against her clitoris, then lick off the juices. Ladle caviar around his penis and eat it off, or make a bikini bottom from caviar and ask him to go down!

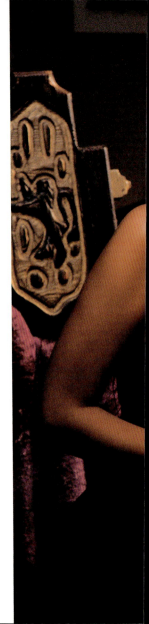

23

What's in the Fridge?

You'll never look at a melon, a cucumber, or a raspberry the same way again after you play this naughty game.

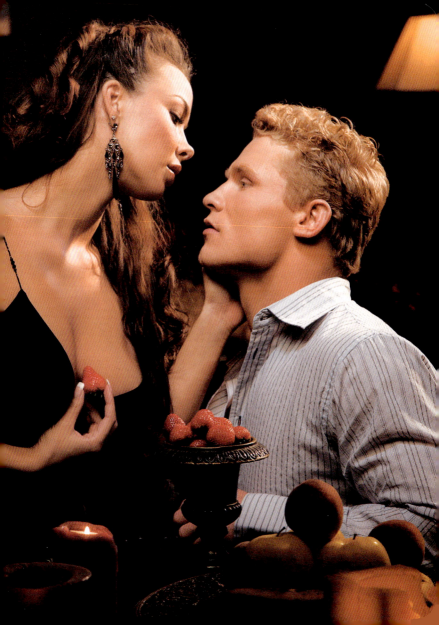

The Sexy Setup

Tell your lover you have a hankering to play with some new toys, but they're all stored right in the fridge.

Rules & Tools

Buy a few cucumbers and scrub them clean (or cover them with a condom). Wash and dry some strawberries or raspberries. Have a honeydew melon and some bologna on hand.

Playing the Game

Sweet and safe: Use the strawberries or raspberries to decorate your nipples, belly button, and genitals, then ask your lover to find the fruit. If you're feeling really bold, hide a few berries in your labia and ask him to eat you out.

Hot and spicy: Use the clean cucumber as a dildo. Ask your lover to apply lubrication and "do me with the cuke," or use a smaller variety for anal sex on either of you.

Up the Ante

- Cut a round hole in one end of a honeydew melon and scoop out a little flesh. Put the melon in the micro-wave for a few minutes, cool slightly and then squirt in some baby oil; ask to watch as your lover gets off with the melon.

- Take a piece of bologna and put it in the microwave for a few seconds, test the temperature, then wrap it around his penis and give him a hand job he'll never forget. Be sure to lick up the "mayo" he makes before you eat the bologna.

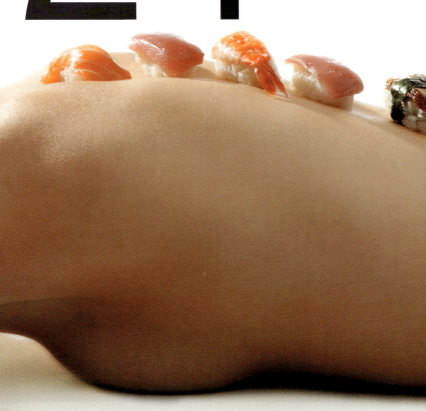

24

Naked Sushi

This sensuous game of eating sushi off your naked body, called *nyotaimori*, originated in Japan, but you can play it right at home—just have your chopsticks ready!

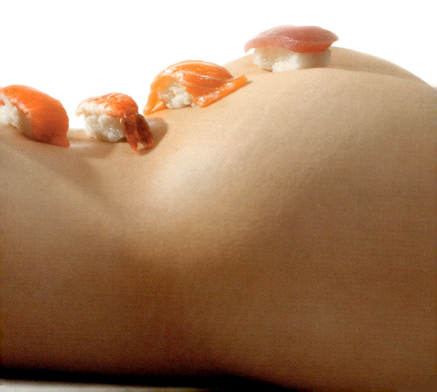

The Sexy Setup

Tell your lover you're serving up "naked sushi" for him tonight and you'll be his private Geisha girl. Arrange a time for your lover to arrive for his meal.

Rules & Tools

You'll need several props for decoration, and you may need a friend to help you with the final assembly. Gather together orchids or other tropical flowers; large tropical or banana leaves; a pair of scallop shells; orange, lemon, or lime slices; and field greens or other exotic-looking vegetables for embellishment. You'll also need an assortment of freshly made sushi and a bottle of sake (Japanese rice wine).

Playing the Game

Sweet and safe: Position yourself on a long counter or dining room table and turn the lights down low. Arrange the scallop shells to cover your nipples, then artfully arrange the flowers, leaves, embellishments, and sushi all over your body.

When your lover arrives, allow him to eat his dinner, delight in your body, and stimulate or tickle you with a chopstick while you try to lie perfectly still.

Hot and spicy: *Wakamezake,* also called seaweed sake, involves letting him drink sake from your naked body. Position yourself sitting up, then close your legs tight enough that the triangle between your thighs and pubic area forms a cup. Ask your lover to pour sake down your chest into this triangle and drink the sake from there. The name comes from the idea that the woman's pubic hair in the sake resembles soft seaweed floating in the sea.

Up the Ante

- Dress like a Japanese sex worker and try *sumata* (which loosely translates to bare crotch). This technique, which involves rubbing your thighs and labia against your lover's penis until he comes, is popular in Japanese brothels and massage parlors where intercourse is forbidden.

- Seek out exhibits of Japanese erotica, called *shunga,* and try the positions at home.

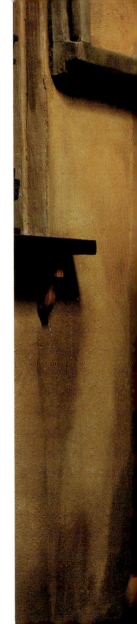

25

Peppermint Tingler

Use the flavor of mint to spice up your sex life with this erotic game.

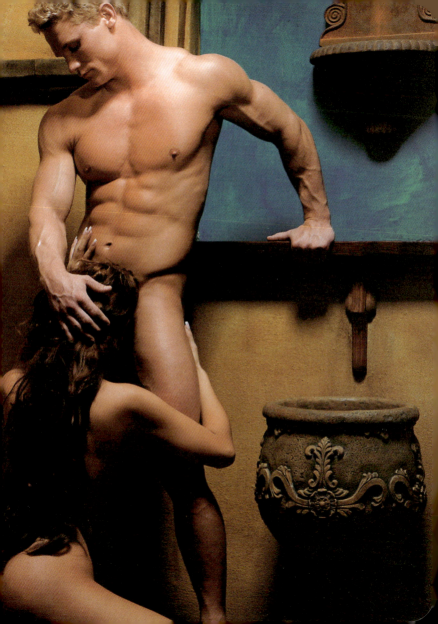

The Sexy Setup

Tell your lover you've planned a minty game with plenty of cool sensations.

Rules & Tools

Buy your favorite flavor of Altoid mints. Pour two glasses of peppermint schnapps, or, if you don't drink, a small glass of cinnamon or minty mouthwash.

Playing the Game

Sweet and safe: Chew some of the Altoids before giving your lover a blow job, or ask your lover to eat Altoids before going down on you. The tingling sensation you feel in your mouth when you chew these mints will intensify the sensation of oral sex for your partner.

Hot and spicy: Tip your glasses to one another and take a small sip of the schnapps. Run your tongues around one another's lips, then slowly move your mouth down your lover's body, leaving a minty cool trail across his skin. Ask your lover to circle your nipples with his minty tongue. Let it pool in your belly button, and then have him lap it out.

Trace a path all the way to his penis. Once you reach your lover's genitals, take another small sip—just enough so that you don't swallow it or drop a whole mouthful over your sweetie's privates. As you slip your mouth over his penis, let the liqueur or mouthwash drip down his shaft. The tingly sensation will drive him wild. If your lover does the same to you, tell him to be especially careful when letting the liqueur drip onto your clitoris and labia, and never let the liqueur or mouthwash get inside your vagina. (Clean yourselves off before having intercourse.)

Up the Ante

- Chew a few Altoids, or take a sip of schnapps, then explore your lover's backside and/or give him or her a rim job. If you want to intensify the sensation, introduce an ice cube for an unexpected combination of ice and spice.

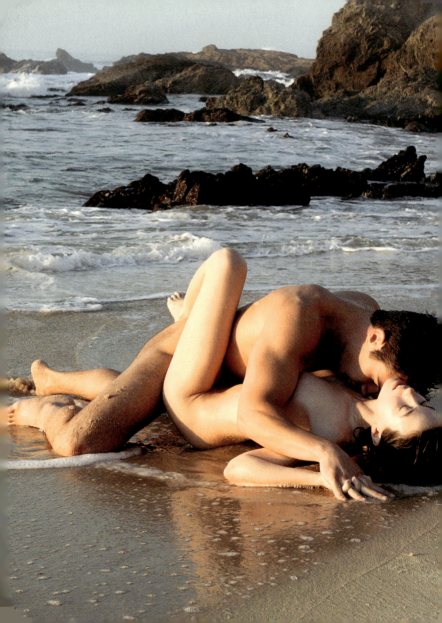

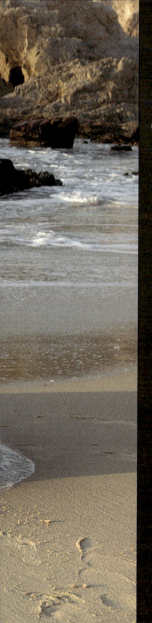

CHAPTER 3

The Great Outdoors

Love the outdoors? Love to have sex? Why not combine the two with this set of fresh-air games. Whether you're frolicking in the woods, masturbating on moss, or making love seaside, Mother Nature offers an endless assortment of settings for naughty games and fun. Just be careful not to get into trouble with the law!

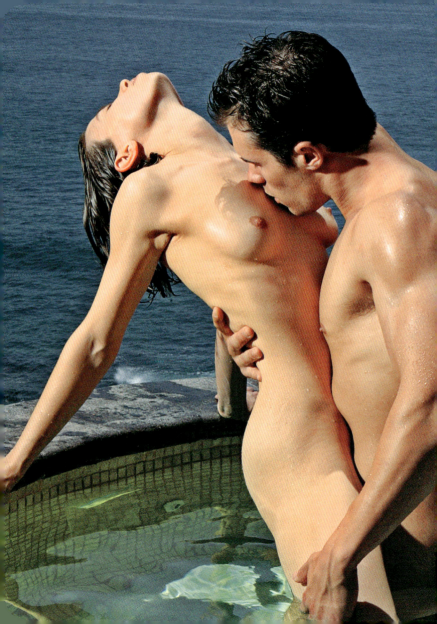

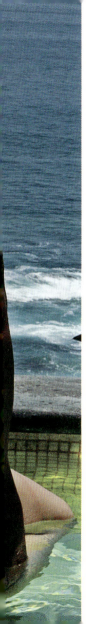

26

Summer Lovin'—
Kiddie-Pool Style

Here's a naughty summertime game that will
heat you up—and cool you down!

The Sexy Setup

Tell your lover just how hot it is outside, but that you have the perfect way to cool things off *and* have a taste of summer fun.

Rules & Tools

Buy yourself a large blow-up kiddie pool (if you don't already have one) and a few bottles of mineral oil (which is not latex friendly). Pour the oil into the pool before you fill it with water. Purchase some children's "water wings" and have Vaseline nearby.

Playing the Game

Sweet and safe: Have your lover kneel and sit on his heels while you lie flat with your head on the opposite edge. Have your lover lift your hips up so they're above the water, then move together to create your own waves!

Hot and spicy: Buy your lover a pair of "water wings" (the kind that little kids wear when they're learning to swim). Blow up the wings, then coat the inside with Vaseline. Move the wing up and down on your lover's penis until he comes!

Up the Ante

- Get out the water pistols, but fill them with wine or champagne. The first person to soak the other gets licked clean.

- Give your lover a water orgasm: Tie your lover to a beach chair, then use a stream of water from the hose or squirt gun to get her off!

- Get out the kid's slip and slide, turn on the hose, and have your lover slip into you while you slide down his shaft.

27

Lakeshore Loving

Who among us hasn't imagined a sexy interlude on the grass next to our favorite skinny-dipping spot?

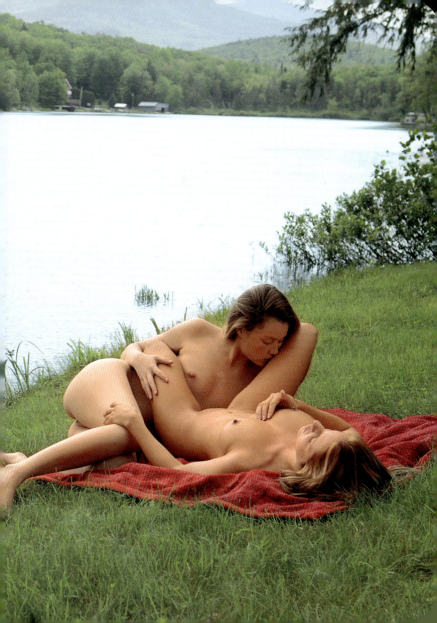

The Sexy Setup

Tell your lover you'd like to go swimming (or skinny-dipping) and you have the perfect game for after your dip.

Rules & Tools

Bring along a blanket or plenty of beach towels for creating a soft bed (don't forget the massage oil!). Make sure you've found a spot where you won't be discovered— or pump up the adrenaline by choosing a spot where you just might get caught!

Playing the Game

Sweet and safe: Play a game of hide-and-seek in the woods near your lake. Whenever you find your lover, remove a piece of his or her clothing. The winner (whoever stays dressed the longest) gets to issue his or her favorite sexy command.

Hot and spicy: Tie your lover to a tree (facing forward or backward) and force him or her to submit to your every directive. Try teasing him by tracing a small twig up his thighs or dipping a smooth stone in massage oil and running it over his buttocks. Or take it up a notch and spank him using a switch made from a branch.

Up the Ante

- Coat yourselves liberally with suntan lotion (or get wet in the lake) and have an outdoor wrestling match. If your lover is taller or heavier than you, then make it fair by tying one arm behind his back or binding his feet together. The object of the game? To get the best of three falls onto your lakeside love bed.

- Find a secluded spot near a waterfall and make love under the waterfall or with the mist swirling all around you. Alternatively, look for sensuous outdoor locations for making love, such as in a cave, in the middle of a field, in the rain, under a canopy of leaves, or on a bed of moss.

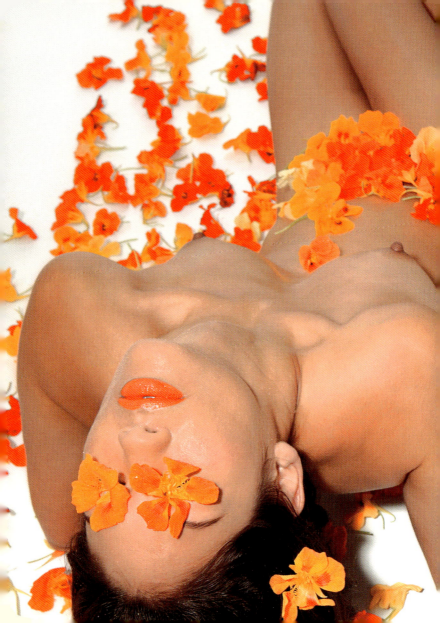

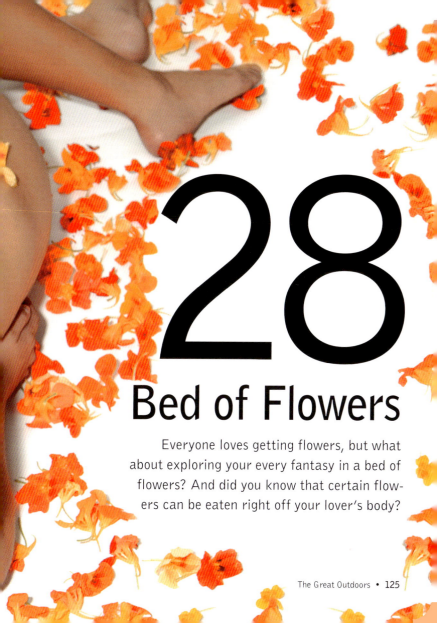

28

Bed of Flowers

Everyone loves getting flowers, but what about exploring your every fantasy in a bed of flowers? And did you know that certain flowers can be eaten right off your lover's body?

The Sexy Setup

Tell your lover you have a soft and sensuous game that's just right for a warm, sunny day in the garden.

Rules & Tools

If you can't find a bed of flowers for your game, you can make your own in a private spot outdoors. Simply purchase two dozen organically grown roses and take the flowers apart one by one to create a bed of petals. Other beautiful (and edible) flowers include organically grown violets and nasturtium (pictured). For the hot and spicy version of the game, be sure to bring along some honey.

Playing the Game

Sweet and safe: Disrobe your lover in a sensuous way, then have him or her lie down naked on the bed of flowers. Brush the blossoms or petals all over his or her body. Gently caress the base of the throat with the softest petals, then use the blossoms to trace a path from the throat to the nipples, belly, shoulders, buttocks, or thighs.

Hot and spicy: Create a ritual-like setting and adorn your lover's body with blossoms and petals, then add in swirls or dabs of honey. Tell her you're a bee looking for nectar and she must lie perfectly still while you eat, suck, or nibble the petals and honey away.

Up the Ante

- Hide the petals or blossoms in your crevices and ask your lover to eat his way out of the garden.

- Find a field of wildflowers and make love with full abandon. Only the birds will hear your cries of pleasure!

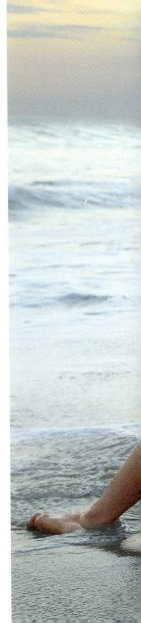

29

Sex on the Beach

All you need for this naughty series of games is your own secluded beach . . . and a little imagination!

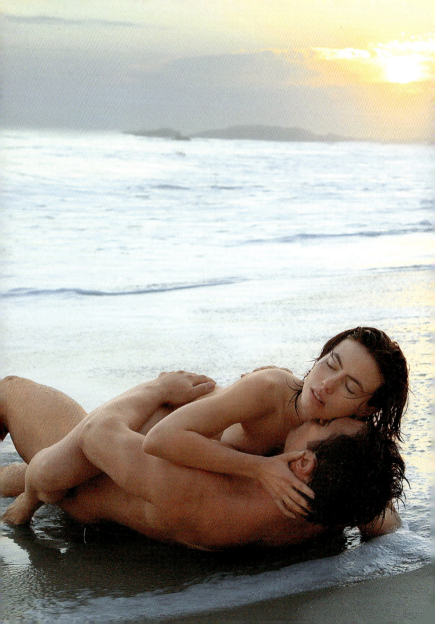

The Sexy Setup

Tell your lover you have a day or evening's worth of fun planned for the seashore.

Rules & Tools

Be sure to bring along all your beach tools, including a waterproof vibrator, spray bottle, sponge, waterproof lubricants, and shovel and pail.

Playing the Game

Sweet and safe: Sculpt each other's naked bodies out of sand, using your own body as a model, or make sexy sand prints by lying down and molding the sand to the contours of your body. Use your shovel to dig out a hole for sitting, then ask your lover to sit in the hole while you climb onto his lap.

Hot and spicy: Pretend you are Aphrodite, goddess of love, beauty, and sexual pleasure. (She was born when Cronus castrated his father, Uranus, and threw his genitals into the ocean!) Adorn yourself in scallop shells and a necklace of seaweed. Ask your lover to lie on the beach, then crawl or emerge out of the ocean like a mermaid come alive. Worship his body by kissing him all over, teasing his inner thighs with your seaweed, and presenting him with the ultimate gift: a wet and sandy blow job or suntan lotion–lubricated hand job.

Up the Ante

- Ask your lover to bury you naked with sand, but leave your nipples, buttocks, or genitals and clitoris uncovered for naughty teasing and pleasuring.

- Make love on the shoreline with the waves crashing against you. Try matching the rhythm of the waves to your thrusts.

- Book a stay in an underwater hotel for a night of unforgettably wet adventures.

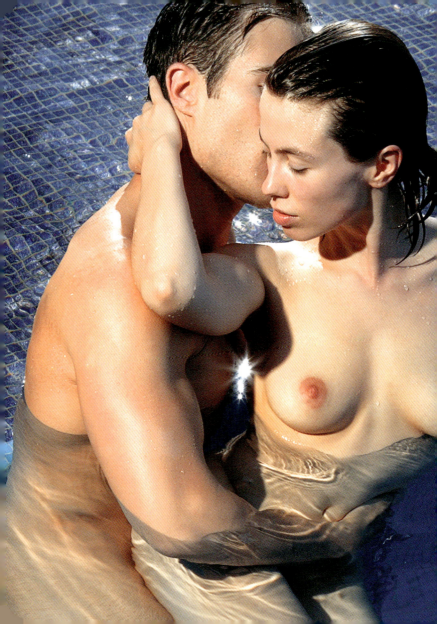

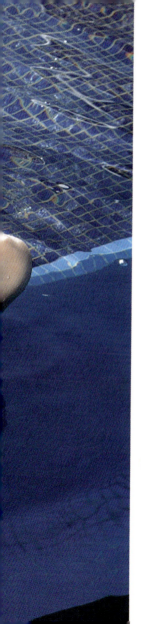

30
Poolside Pussy

Forget the images of screaming kids and lifeguards. These X-rated pool games are for adults only and best played under the stars.

The Sexy Setup

Tell your lover you have a nighttime poolside rendezvous planned, no bathing suit needed!

Rules & Tools

All you need is private and secluded access to a swimming pool and a clear, star-filled night for this naughty night-time game.

Playing the Game

Sweet and safe: Try this erotic version of "Marco Polo" (bathing suit optional!). Hop into the pool and blindfold your lover. Tell him he must find you based on your moans of pleasure (loud for close, soft for far). Once he finds you, reward your lover with a wet and watery kiss, an under-water groping session, or a quick finger in the anus. Then switch roles!

Hot and spicy: Try some watery lovemaking positions using the pool to your advantage. Stay in the shallow end of the pool, and have your lover lean against the wall of the pool for added support. Wrap your legs around his waist and have him penetrate you. Hold on to the edge of the pool if needed. Alternatively, try the ladder: Face the ladder, holding the bars, and have your lover enter you from behind. Or try having him kneel on the step, and you straddle his lap.

Up the Ante

- Challenge your partner to fully remove his or her bathing suit in a public swimming pool and get it back on without anyone noticing.

- Sit naked at the very edge of the pool (or diving board, if he's really strong!) and have your lover pull himself up from underneath to lick and nuzzle your clitoris.

- Try making love on top of an inner tube, air mattress, or other floating pool toy!

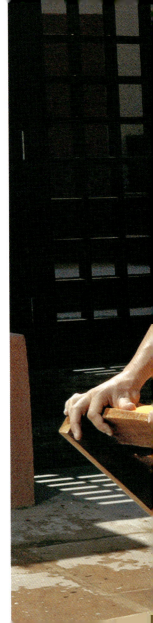

31
Lounge Chair Lovin'

Who says you have to get in the pool
to play this game? Just use the poolside
chairs and tables for props.

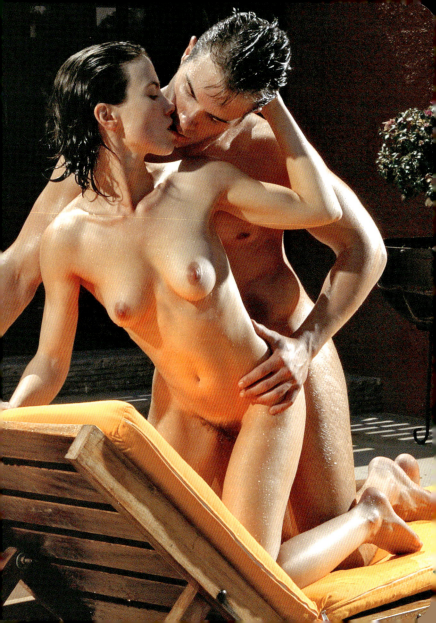

The Sexy Setup

Coax your lover out to the pool, and take a quick dip together to cool off. Then remove his bathing suit for him, slip out of your bikini, and lead him over to the pool deck.

Rules & Tools

Have your lounge chair—and some mineral oil or suntan lotion—ready. Be careful if your lovemaking gets vigorous—some pool furniture may not hold up under heavy thrusting! Better to seek out sturdier pieces (or just pull off the cushions and go for it poolside) to make sure no one falls off the furniture!

Playing the Game

Sweet and safe: Set the chair back to mid-level recline, then lean with your breasts against the chair back and have him tease, taste, and tickle your backside. Ask him to start by kissing the nape of your neck, then trail his tongue down your spine to the small of your back. There's no doubt you'll feel his erection bumping your backside, but make sure he touches your nipples and clitoris to heat you up before he enters you from behind.

Hot and spicy: Have your lover sit or lie down on his favorite lounge chair, then tie his hands and feet to the chair. Start with an all-over body massage using mineral oil or suntan lotion, but wait until he's rock hard before you straddle the chair and ride the waves!

Up the Ante

- Set the chair back to mid-level recline, then lie with your legs dangling over the edge, your genitals right at the edge of the chair. Ask your lover to stand or kneel at the edge of the chair and start exploring you from the feet upward.

- Have your lover stand over the mid-level reclined chair and then lean forward so you can gently spank him with a wet towel.

- Position yourself, facedown, with the lower half of your body on the lounge chair, but your arms on the ground supporting your upper body. Have your lover enter you from behind while grabbing the edge of the chair. Make sure you don't tip over!

- Have him prop you up on the picnic table, or lie side by side in the poolside hammock!

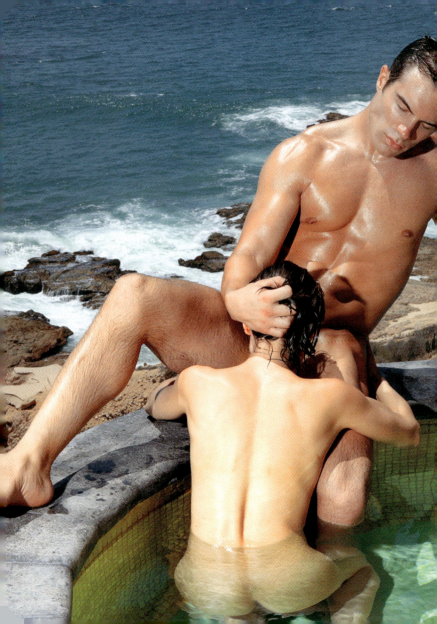

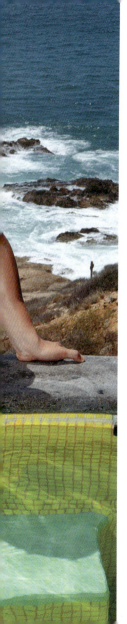

32

Hot Times in the Hot Tub

There's nothing like relaxing in a hot tub to soak away your worries, and everyone knows that a worry-free mind is open for naughty adventures.

The Sexy Setup

Tell your lover you have a nude party planned for the nearest hot tub, and there's one name on the invitation list: HIS!

Rules & Tools

Take care in the hot tub not to slip or submerge your head under water. Remember that water can dry out your genitals, so bring some lubricant along if needed.

Playing the Game

Sweet and safe: Ask your lover to sit on the bench, facing into the tub. Kneel on the bench, with your legs straddling him, before you lower yourself onto his penis. Hold on to the edge of the tub for better support as you raise and lower yourself.

Hot and spicy: Lower yourself onto your lover but face away from him, which will let him gently twist your nipples, stroke your clitoris, or massage your buttocks as you move up and down.

Up the Ante

- Kneel in front of a water jet so it stimulates your clitoris, then ask your lover to enter you from behind for double the fun!

- Have him sit or kneel in front of the water jet so it stimulates his anus. Kiss him passionately while you given him an underwater hand job.

33

Ride the Waves
(in a Boat!)

Whether your lover drives a thirty-foot
motorboat, likes to wave jump on a jet ski,
or prefers quieter waters by paddling a canoe or
kayak, there's plenty of opportunity for naughty
nautical times with these simple games.

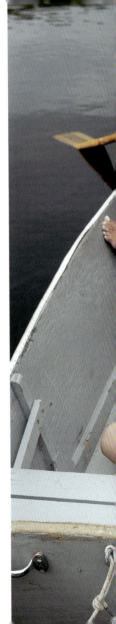

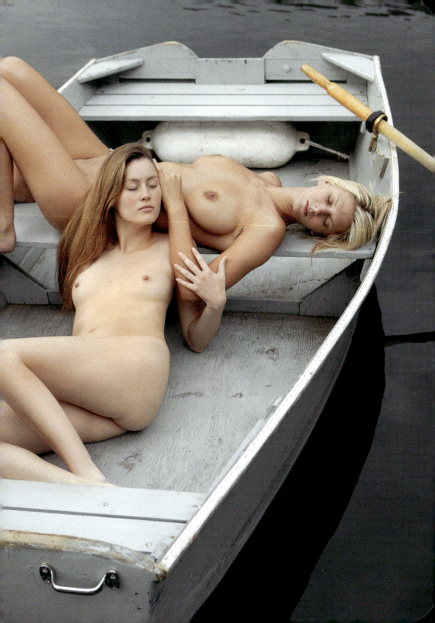

The Sexy Setup

If your lover doesn't own a boat, suggest renting one for a hot summer afternoon. Most marinas will rent motorboats or pontoon boats, and many adventure spots offer kayak, rowboat, or canoe rentals for a small fee. Wear your sexiest bathing suit with a light and airy cover-up, and be sure to bring along lots of lotion for sun protection (or your favorite lubrication, of course!).

Rules & Tools

Let your man drive the boat—chances are he knows how, and it will give him a feeling of power. Make sure you have plenty of gas, a cooler full of beer or wine, a picnic lunch, and some beach blankets or towels.

Playing the Game

Sweet and safe: Take the boat out into the middle of the lake (where you might have more privacy than anchoring near shore), enjoy your picnic, and go for a swim. Once you're back in the boat, offer to help him dry off.

As you rub him down, rub your body up against him suggestively, then gently strip off his bathing suit while stroking his buttocks, penis, and legs. Ease him onto one of the seats, then start kissing him from the neck down. Give him a luscious blow job in time with the gentle lapping of the waves.

Hot and spicy: If you're renting a pontoon boat, the seats and floor give you plenty of space for having sex. This game is even more fun at night, when most boaters have left the lake, and you can chug into a secluded area for some nautical nooky!

Up the Ante

- Take out a rowboat, kayak, or canoe and paddle to a deserted island or beach. Go for a swim, have a bite to eat, then tell your lover you want to play water nymph.

- Have him lie naked in shallow water, then swim out a short distance, turn around, and approach him from under the water. Try to touch, kiss, and stroke his feet, legs, and genitals as much as possible while under the water, then finally work your way up to giving him a blow job or climbing astride!

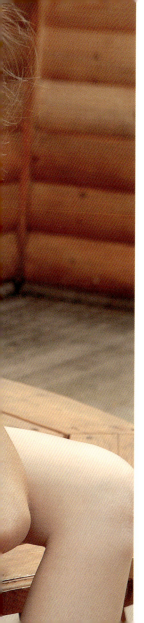

34

Playin' on the Playground

Think the playground is just for kids? Think again! Swings, tunnels, and slides are the perfect props for these adult-only games.

The Sexy Setup

Tell your lover to meet you at the playground after dark for some nighttime nooky.

Rules & Tools

Find a secluded and private playground. Bring flashlights, a bottle of wine, and blankets, if desired.

Playing the Game

Sweet and safe: Act like kids again, but this time do it in your birthday suits. Climb the ladder to the slide, pausing on the rung of your choice to give him a good look at your back view, then slide down the slide and have him kneel at the edge for some quick flicks of his tongue on your clitoris. Or, bring along a flashlight and play hide-and-seek in the dark (clothing optional!).

Hot and spicy: Have him sit on the swing, then you straddle him. Hold on tight! Alternatively, go through the tunnel slide together, side by side. When you get to the bottom, try making love inside the slide, or position yourself at the top of the tube and have him stand in front—your fully exposed genitals should be right at eye (and tongue!) level.

Up the Ante

- Have him tie you spread-eagle to the ladder rungs, then explore every crevice with his hands and tongue. Alternatively, have him tie you backside facing out, then examine all your assets.

- Climb astride the overhead monkey bars with your legs over the bar and your genitals at face level. Ask him to explore your underside using his tongue, fingers, and hands!

- Sit in the swing and have him stimulate your clitoris with his tongue. Push away when the sensation is too strong, then swing back for more oral stimulation until you come!

- Try making love on a trampoline, in a tree house, or on the top bunk of a bunk bed! Remember, you *can* be a kid again when it comes to sexual adventure!

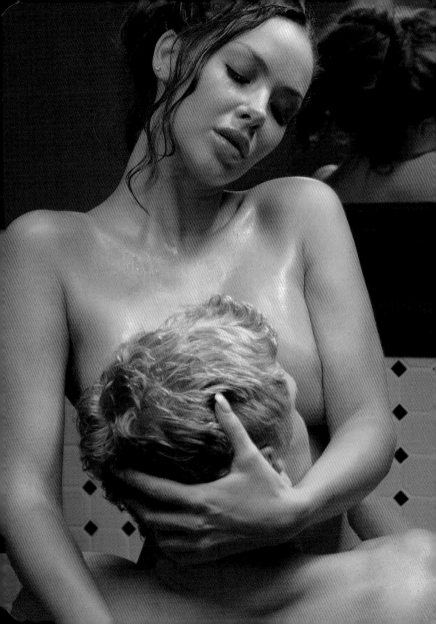

CHAPTER 4

Position Games

Love to try new positions?
Then you've come to the right
place—a whole set of games
revolving around positions
for both intercourse and oral
sex. You're sure to get a workout for all your love muscles
with these randy games!

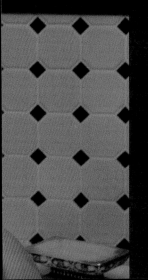

35

Missionary Man

There's nothing wrong with going back to basics from time to time, and this naughty game will remind you of all the traditional positions for intercourse—and the variations that can heighten your pleasure!

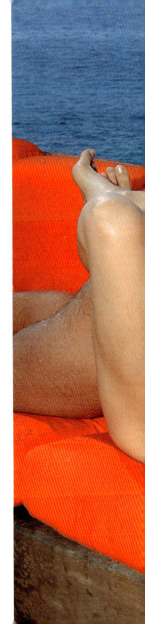

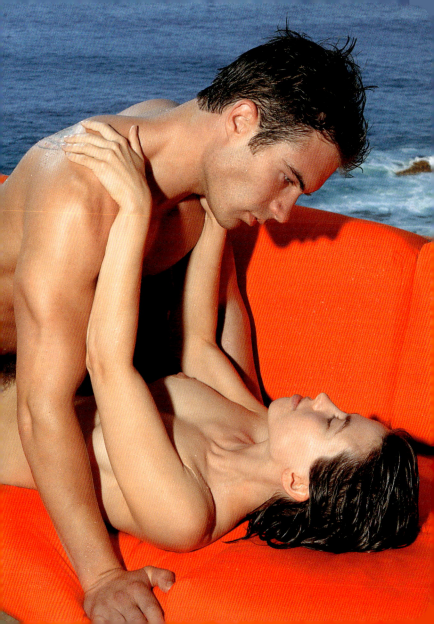

The Sexy Setup

Send your lover a note, and tell her you're a man on a
mission: to explore some new options for penetration.

Rules & Tools

Set a sexy scene, such as in the bedroom, on an outdoor
couch, or on the floor of a private room. Light some candles, dim the lights, and put on some soft music. If you're
playing this game on the floor, put down some soft blankets and toss some pillows around.

Playing the Game

Sweet and safe: Undress your lover one article of clothing after another, taking time to kiss her neck, fondle her
breasts, and massage her buttocks in order to get you both
ready for sex. Have her lie on her back, then you lie on
top of her, with your legs stretched out straight behind you.
Ask her to spread her legs so you can enter her, but then to
stretch her legs out straight in the "clasp position." Have
her pull her legs together to tightly sandwich your penis
and add to the friction.

Hot and spicy: To take it up a notch, have her pull her legs upward and wrap them around your waist. To progress even further (and deepen the penetration!), ask her to pull her legs toward her head and hook her heels on your shoulders. Lock eyes with your lover, then ask her to grab your hindquarters and pull you into her. Alternatively, pin her hands above her head for a feeling of domination.

Up the Ante

- Once her ankles are by your shoulders, ask your lover to move her legs back and forth sideways in the air, squeezing your penis from both sides. This move, called scissors, feels sensational!

- Once you're in the missionary position, turn a full 360 degrees with your penis still inside her. (This will take some practice to prevent your penis from slipping out of her!) Once you're facing her feet, ask her to massage your buttocks while you thrust away.

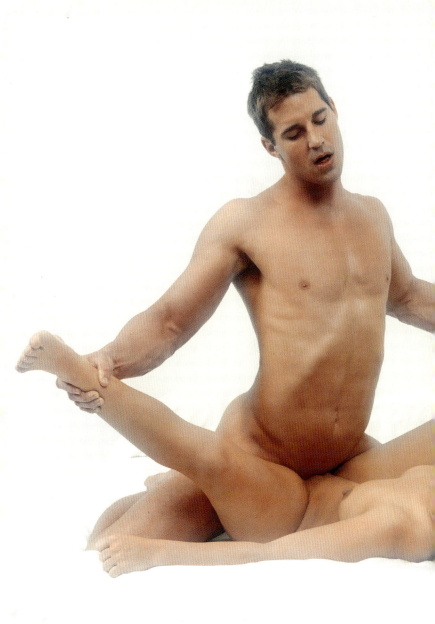

36

Get on Your Knees

Here's a set of positions that will get you on your knees—and praying for more!

The Sexy Setup

Write your lover a note and tell him you had a hot and sexy dream last night, and you're dying to show him what happened in the dream.

Rules & Tools

Set a sexy scene for your game: Buy some new soft blankets for your bed, or dress up in a sexy low-cut dress with your highest heels. Remember, men are stimulated visually, so aim to get him hot before the game even begins!

Playing the Game

Sweet and safe: Lie on your back and have your lover kneel in front of you. Once he's entered you, have him take a firm grip on your ankles and spread your legs as wide as they can comfortably go. Tell him to take a look at his erect penis moving in and out of your vagina—he's sure to be visually stimulated! While your legs are spread wide, touch your clitoris or fondle your nipples for extra pleasure.

Hot and spicy: To progress to the next position, lift one leg and put it on his shoulder, but let the other leg lie flat or wrap it around his waist. Twist your body if needed so he can penetrate you even further. To take it up a notch, reposition yourself so the lowered leg is under your kneeling lover.

Up the Ante

- Twist your body as you lower your leg; your lover is still kneeling, but now he's aligned with your hip and side. Enjoy the new sensations with this action!

- Turn one more time to lie on your stomach with your lover on top of you, his legs straight behind. This is a great position for stimulating your G-spot.

37

In the Lap of Luxury

This intimate and sexy position will surely bring you closer, both emotionally and sexually.

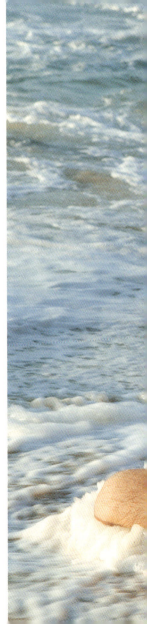

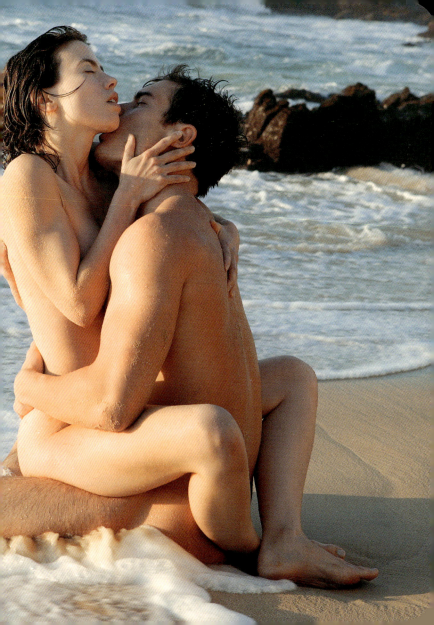

The Sexy Setup

Tell your lover you're in need of some full frontal nudity
and contact, so be prepared for connecting your skin at
every possible point. What's more, you'll do all the work
while sitting on his lap.

Rules & Tools

All of these positions are done with both of you facing
each other, so there's plenty of opportunity for making
eye contact, licking his nipples, or having him fondle
your breasts.

Playing the Game

Sweet and safe: Undress your lover in a slow and sensuous manner, then have him remove your clothing, all the while kissing your neck and breasts and rubbing his hands up and down your backside. Once you're both hot and wet, ask your lover to sit cross-legged. You should sit down on his lap, facing him, while inserting his penis into your vagina. Straddle his legs and wrap your legs around his back, then rub the front of your bodies together while you experience the sensations of shallow but tight penetration.

Hot and spicy: Lean back with one arm and hook one leg over his shoulder to change the angle of penetration, or slowly lean both arms backward, exposing your breasts for fondling or your clitoris for stimulation.

Up the Ante

- Ask your lover to stretch out his legs while you sit or lean back. To deepen the penetration, rest your legs on your partner's shoulders instead of wrapping them around his waist and lean back on your arms. For a sexy variation on this position that gives him full view of your naked torso, lie completely down on your back and lock your ankles behind his neck.

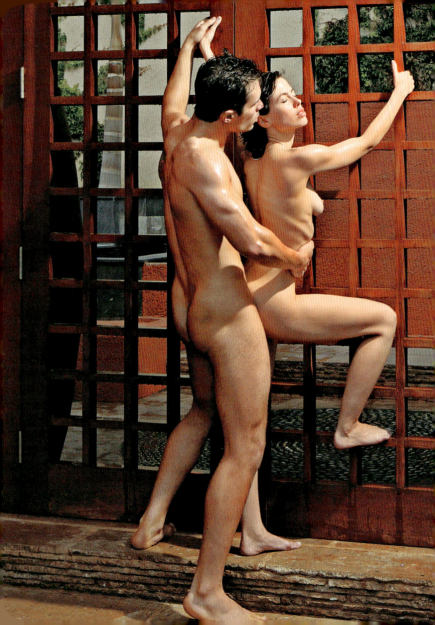

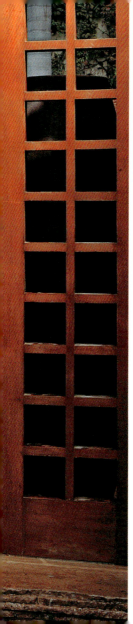

38

Prop Me Up
(and Drive It Home!)

This is the perfect sex game for locations where there's no room for lying down, such as a quickie in a restroom, a sexy encounter in the front hall, or a racy rendezvous in the closet while the kids watch a movie!

The Sexy Setup

Tell your lover you have a game that's sure to get a standing ovation. Mention that you've always wanted to enter her from behind, with her leg propped on a chair, or that you know a certain doorway that's perfect for face-to-face entry!

Rules & Tools

Bring along some lubrication, and perhaps a stool or chair for support.

Playing the Game

Sweet and safe: Undress each other slowly and sensuously, then find a place to prop your lover against the wall, facing away from you. Stroke her breasts and rub your hands down her belly, then slowly lift one of her legs up, prop it on a stool or small chair, and enter her from behind. The beauty of this position is that you can fondle her breasts, finger her clitoris, or gently bite the nape of her neck while you have intercourse!

Hot and spicy: Lean her against a wall or doorway, but have her face you so you can kiss her passionately, gently nip at her neck and shoulders, and run your hands down her backside. Lift one of her legs up, wrapping it around your waist or propping it on a small stool, then stoop slightly so you can enter her from below.

Up the Ante

- Brace yourself against a doorway with your hands on one side and your feet on the opposite side. Ask your lover to straddle you, with her feet on the same side of the doorway as you and her arms on the opposite side.

- Lean against the same doorpost, but invite your lover to climb aboard and hold on to your neck. Brace yourself with your legs while you thrust away!

39

Spoonful of Lovin'

Just like a spoonful of sugar, this position game is
sweet and easy. Perfect for a lazy Sunday morning!

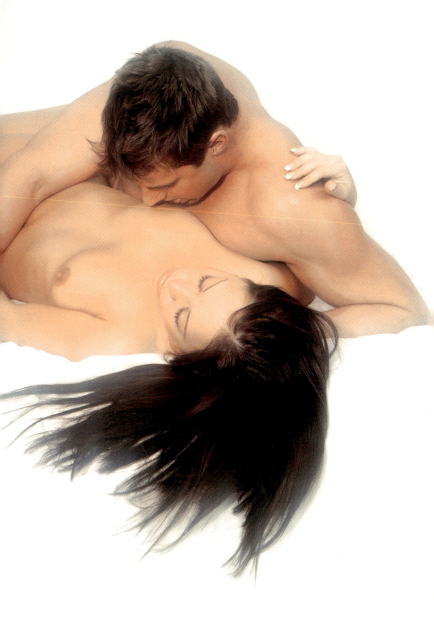

The Sexy Setup

You're cuddling in bed, and your lover isn't quite awake. Come up to her from behind, spooning against her backside, fondle her breasts, and whisper in her ear until she wakes up.

Rules & Tools

This is a slow and sensuous position—so take your time and enjoy stimulating your lover while you enter her from behind.

Playing the Game

Sweet and safe: Start by having your lover lie on her side, then rub your hands all over her front side. Fondle her breasts, gently squeeze her nipples, rub your hands longingly down her belly and over her hips, and then work your way over to her clitoris. Get her hot and wet, then gently part her legs slightly and slip inside.

Hot and spicy: Stimulate her clitoris and softly kiss and nip the back of her neck while you gently and slowly thrust away. To draw out the game, pull out of her occasionally, kiss her fully and deeply, then slide back inside and continue the action.

Up the Ante

- If you're ready for more action, flip her over and take her doggie style!

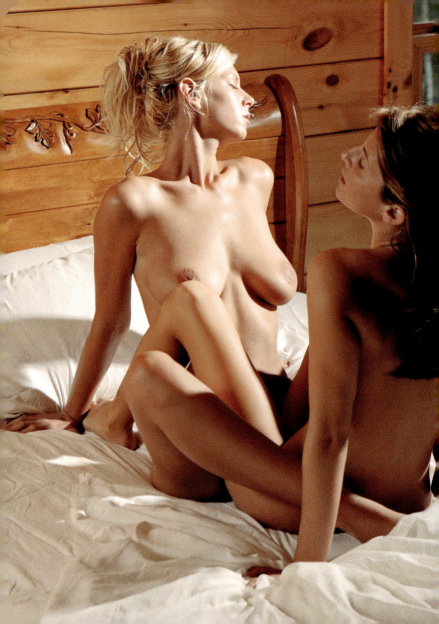

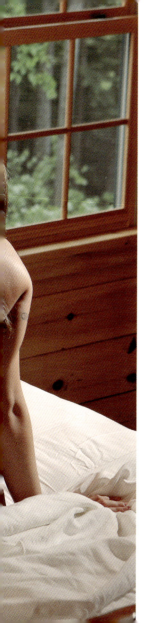

40

Scissors
of Love

This is a game designed for a pair of women, but it can also be modified for you and your male lover if it turns you on!

The Sexy Setup

Tell your female lover you're wondering what it will feel like to sit clit to clit, together! If your lover is male, tell him you have a jigsaw puzzle that needs assembling.

Rules & Tools

No real rules or tools here—just the desire to try a new and interesting position!

Playing the Game

Sweet and safe (for two women): Start things out slow, caressing each other, kissing, and gently removing each other's clothing. Once things are properly heated up (and you're both naked), move slowly into position: Scissor your legs, then scoot toward each other until your genitals touch. Gently bump and grind your genitals together for stimulation or orgasm; if you can't come without direct stimulation, unwind and take turns using your lips, tongue, or fingers to slowly caress and tease each other to orgasm.

Hot and spicy (for a man and a woman): Take your time with your foreplay, making sure your lover is rock hard before you move into position. Curl up on your side, exposing your genitals to your lover. He slides toward you, legs scissoring each other, in order to complete the jigsaw puzzle.

Up the Ante

- For two women: Try the male/female version of this position, but use a finger to stimulate your lover anally. Or, once she's in the curled position, take out your dildo and penetrate her while you rub together, clit to clit!

- While sitting in the sweet and safe position, insert a two-headed dildo into both of you and slide back and forth together.

41

Cowgirl and Bucking Bronco

Who doesn't love a little game of ride 'em, cowgirl? This time the lady leads the way and dictates just how much she likes bucking and deep penetration.

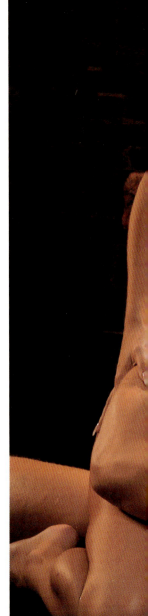

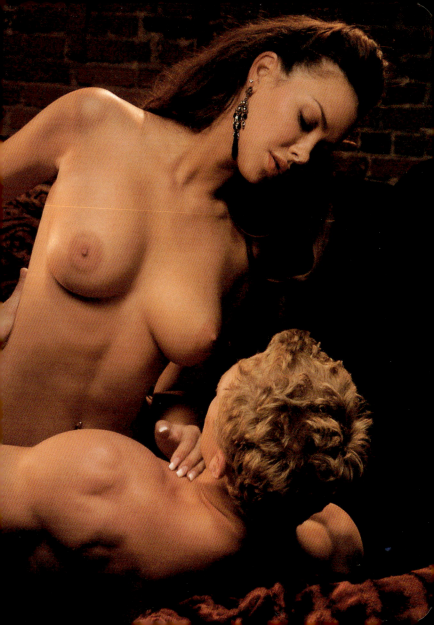

The Sexy Setup

Tell your lover it's your turn to control the pleasure.
He should lie back and enjoy the ride (as well as the
scenery!).

Rules & Tools

All of these positions involve the woman on top while he
lies down. Sometimes this amount of deep penetration can
be intense, so vary the angle, the tempo, or the depth of
thrusting to maximize your pleasure.

Playing the Game

Sweet and safe: Have your lover lie on his back, then
lick his thighs, suck his penis, and fondle his buttocks
in order to get him hard. Use lubrication if needed, then
straddle him, face to face, and insert his penis into you.
Place your hands on his chest for support, and ask him
to fondle your breasts or pinch your nipples while you
rise up and down.

Hot and spicy: Try the straddling action from a different starting point for even deeper penetration. Have him kneel, sitting back on his legs. Slowly sit down on his lap, straddling him again and tucking your feet behind you and onto his knees. Put your arms around his neck for support and have him hold your back for better control.

Up the Ante

- Straddle your lover, but face away from him (giving him full view of your backside). This is a good position for G-spot stimulation.

- Have your lover lie down, then lower yourself onto him sideways. Ask him to stimulate your clitoris while you surf his wave.

- After you're done riding your bronco, let him taste his own secretions: Slide upward so he can stimulate your clitoris with his mouth and tongue. Raise or lower your body, or rock forward and backward, to increase your pleasure.

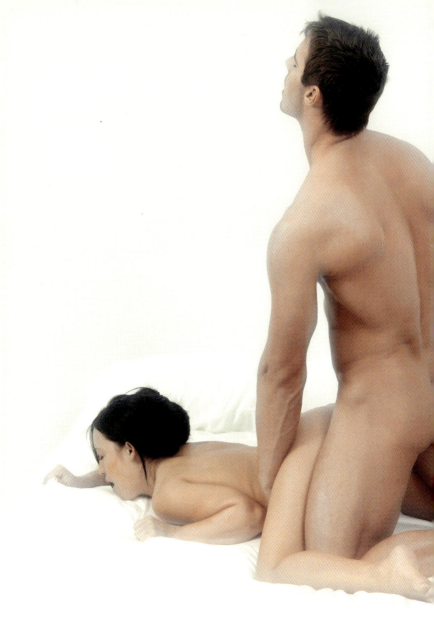

42

Doggie Style

You've seen dogs do it, and maybe
even cats, rabbits, or squirrels.
Now it's your turn to act
like an animal!

The Sexy Setup

Tell your lover you have a position that will give her the deep penetration she's been craving—and you'll do all the work!

Rules & Tools

This position is best suited for a soft surface (to protect your knees). If you're not on a bed or other soft surface, use a pillow or blanket under your knees.

Playing the Game

Sweet and safe: Arouse your lover in the way you know best. Once she's hot and wet, ask her to kneel on all fours. Kneel upright behind her and gently enter her from behind, then grab a hold of her hips and thrust away.

Hot and spicy: Try the Dutch Doggy: While you penetrate your lover, have her stretch out one leg, then the other in a windmill motion. You'll be amazed at the intense penetration that's possible as you share this canine variation!

Up the Ante

- For a dominant variation on traditional doggie style, have your lover lean on a chair or the bed, then pin her arms down and give her every inch of what you've got!

- Try the Basset Hound: Have your lover lie on her stomach with her legs tucked under her and her shoulders and face on the ground. Kneel behind her, but shift your knees to either side of her buttocks. You'll both need flexible hips for this position, but the effort is worth it!

- Swap positions, so now you're on your hands and knees. Let her kneel behind you, then reach around to massage your penis with one hand and fondle your testicles with her other!

43

Classic 69

Everyone knows the meaning of 69,
but do you know all the different
variations of this classic position
for oral sex?

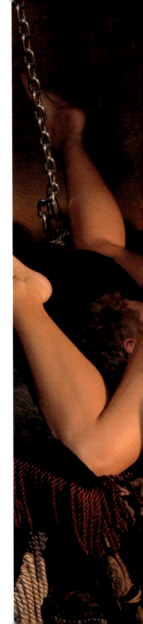

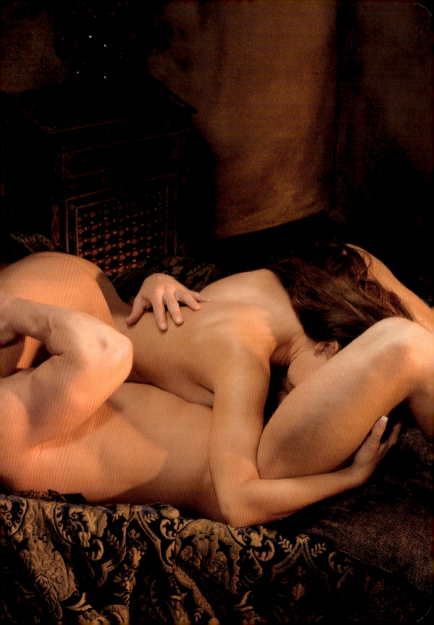

The Sexy Setup

This is an easy game to pitch to your lover—you'll both get your share of oral pleasure! Tell her you're going for a ride on Route 69, you're going to play a game of 6s and 9s, or ask her to pick a number between 68 and 70 and guess what's coming!

Rules & Tools

This game takes a little concentration, as you're going to lick, suck, and use your tongue to give him (or her) a mind-blowing orgasm while he (or she) returns the favor.

Playing the Game

Sweet and safe: Lie side by side with your lover, and rest your head on her inner thigh. (She can rest her head on your inner thigh.) Imagine her genital area as a flower that you are slowly and gently going to open up using your tongue and lips. Gently tease and kiss around her outer labia, using your fingers to part them slightly. Use your tongue to feel for her inner lips, then flick her clitoris once or twice. Insert a finger into her vagina or her anus, then slowly increase the intensity and duration of your tongue on her clitoris. Use your fingers to gently expose the clit completely and use gentle laps of your tongue to bring her to orgasm!

Hot and spicy: Try these variations on the Classic 69: Have your lover lie on top of you, facing your feet. Prop a pillow under your head so you can reach her genitals without straining your neck. Alternatively, lie on top of her and bury your head between her thighs. Your penis will dangle right over her mouth!

Up the Ante

- Try the Curled 69: Curl into a tucked position for a tighter, more intimate version of the Classic 69.

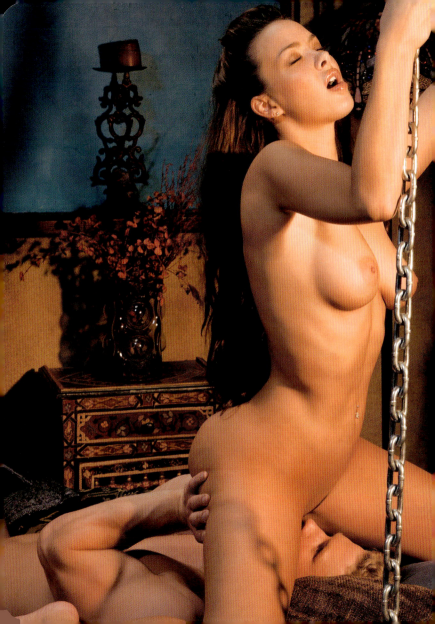

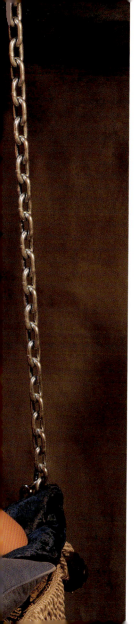

44

Sit on My Face

Come sit on my face—who hasn't heard
that enticing line? Now you can turn it
into a game that's sure to keep her
coming back for more!

The Sexy Setup

Tell your lover you have a game where she gets to sit—
right on the pleasure dome (your mouth)!

Rules & Tools

If you're not on a bed or other soft surface, put a blanket
or pillow under her knees. Explain to her that she's in
control—while you're there to pleasure her orally, she
can control the intensity by moving up and down on your
tongue. If she needs something to hold on to, position yourselves so she can lean her hands against the wall or hold
on to the swing (as shown). For the hot and spicy version of
the game, keep a butt plug or other anal device nearby.

Playing the Game

Sweet and safe: Have your lover kneel above your face,
facing you, while you explore every inch of what's right
in front of you. Start by kissing her inner thighs and taking in the smell and taste of her vulva. Give her genitals
long, slow, and wet kisses, then introduce your tongue for
exploring her labia, crevices, and clitoris. Find a rhythm
she likes and bring her to a mind-blowing orgasm!

Hot and spicy: Have your lover kneel above your face, facing away from you, while you explore her genitals and backside. Use the same techniques as above, but don't restrict your kisses and tongue exploration to her labia and clitoris; run your tongue from her vagina to her anus and back again, all the while gently massing her buttocks. Put a finger or two inside her vagina and play with her G-spot, or introduce a butt plug or other anal device and insert that for triple stimulation!

Up the Ante

- Swap roles: Have her lie down, then kneel in front of her so your penis is right in front of her mouth (she may need a pillow or two to get the angle right). Have her hold your penis with one hand and explore your backside with the other; she might fondle your testicles, insert a finger into your anus, or just lightly trace her fingertips along your perineum.

45

Seat of Honor

Treat your lover like the queen she is,
and give her the seat of honor.
She'll never stray far from
your kingdom!

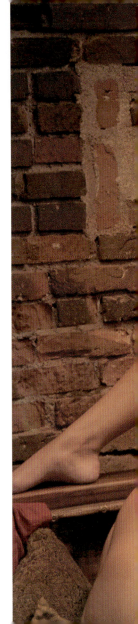

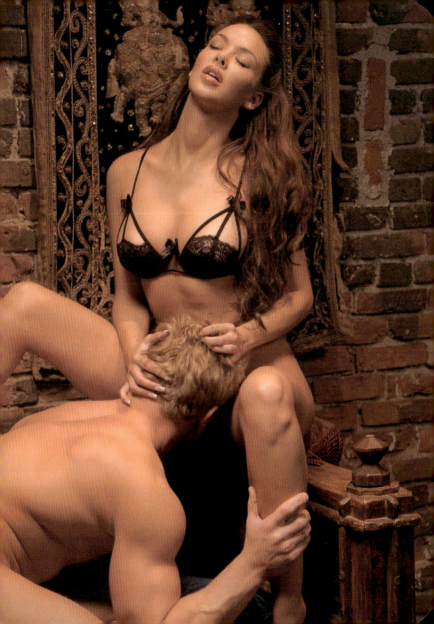

The Sexy Setup

Tell your lover you're her adoring knight, and you want to treat her like a queen. Specifically, you have a seat of honor that promises hours of pleasure!

Rules & Tools

This is all about pleasuring your lover, so be prepared to spend some time on your knees, exploring all her most glorious treasures! If you want to get into role-playing, dress like a squire or knight, and ask her to dress like a queen. Then set up a throne by draping furs or velvet over a chair and giving her a crown.

Playing the Game

Sweet and safe: Lead your lover to her throne, perhaps blindfolded so she doesn't know what awaits her. Slowly and seductively remove her clothing, or if you're playing a game of adulterous royal love, lift up her skirts and bury your face in her privates. Lick and tease her inner thighs, then use your hands, mouth, lips, or tongue to give her an orgasm befitting a queen!

Hot and spicy: In this scenario, pretend you are a foreign knight who has taken the queen hostage. Your duty: not to hurt her, but to pleasure her beyond her wildest dreams. Lead her to her throne, but then tie her hands to the chair. Spread her legs and tie her legs to the chair as well. Now she's your captive, and you can tease her until she screams for mercy—or moans with pleasure!

Up the Ante

- Put together a "Royal Tool Kit" full of her favorite sex toys and props, then use them one by one while she's strapped to the chair. Use an anal vibrator to stimulate her backside while you lick her clitoris, or bring her to orgasm manually while you penetrate her with a dildo.

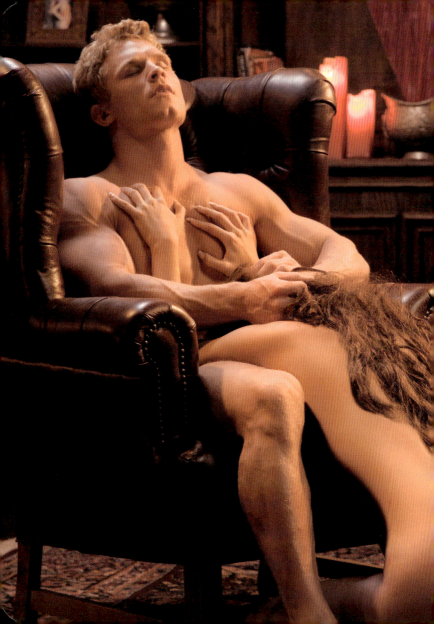

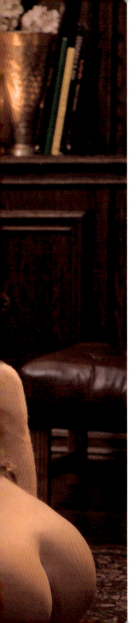

46

At Your Service

Ladies, it's your turn to service your king: Get on your knees and get ready for pleasuring his majesty!

The Sexy Setup

Tell your lover you have a plan: He gets to be king for the
night. You're the mistress he's plucked from the royal
court or the lowly servant who must always serve her
master, and serve him well!

Rules & Tools

Set up a throne by draping furs or velvet over a couch.
Dress in a maiden's dress (with no undergarments) and
buy him a royal-looking cape, crown, or coat.

Playing the Game

Sweet and safe: Lead your lover to his throne, and ask
him where he most likes to be kissed. Start kissing him
there, but then take your kisses to his neck, his chest, his
belly, and downward. Kiss him all over, but avoid his
genitals until he orders you to touch him *there*. Then suck,
nibble, and bite your way around until he orders you to
make him come. Follow his orders, naturally!

Hot and spicy: Before you sit him down and begin stimulating him, sit on his lap and hand feed him grapes or let him sip champagne. Treat him royally, showering him with affection while he relaxes and unwinds. Surprise him suddenly by tying him to the chair (a short struggle will turn you both on!) and removing just enough of his clothes to reveal his genitals. Although he's king, he's also your prisoner, and you intend to draw out your pleasurable torture. Undress seductively and tease him in a sexy manner, all the while knowing he cannot touch you. When he's sufficiently turned on, bring him to orgasm in whatever way you please.

Up the Ante

- If you enjoy role-playing, there are plenty of famous kings, queens, and lovers you can reenact, from Cleopatra and Mark Antony to Henry VIII and his mistresses.

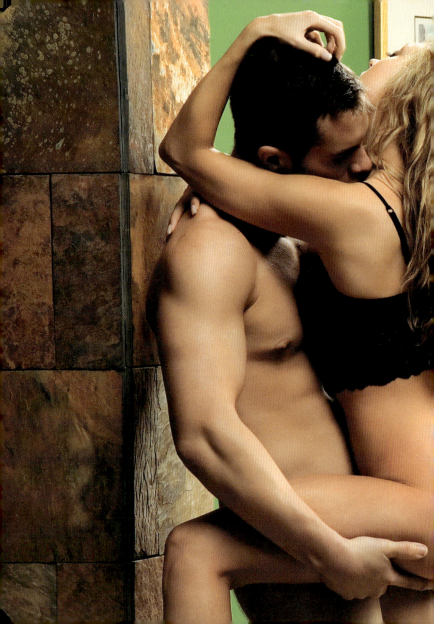

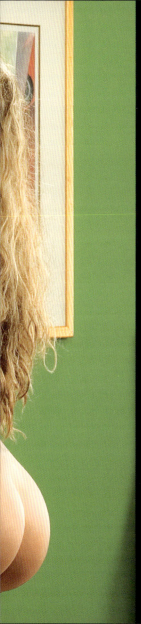

CHAPTER 5

Forbidden Territories

If you've always wanted to join the Mile High Club, have sex in a furniture store, or get it on in the department store dressing room, you'll love the naughty games in this fun-filled section. Just remember to work up a creative excuse beforehand in case you get caught!

47

Going Down, Anyone?

What could be more exciting than sex in an elevator—and if you're lucky, the walls will be padded for softer pushing (and absorbing the sound of his groans of pleasure . . .).

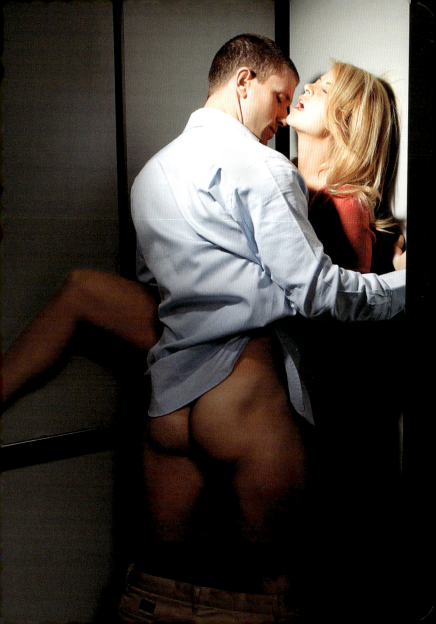

The Sexy Setup

Set up a rendezvous ahead of time by sending your lover a sexy email or text message. Tell him what time which floor he should be waiting on. Be sure to wear a skirt (without undergarments!) for easy access.

Rules & Tools

Research your elevator beforehand and test the "stop" button—pushing it between floors may cause an alarm to ring, which is sure to dampen the mood. Older elevator models or freight elevators are more likely to have a "stop" button that lets you halt the elevator between floors. Be on the lookout for a security camera and be aware that sound carries well in an elevator shaft.

Playing the Game

Sweet and safe: As soon as your lover gets on the elevator, have him push (and hold) the stop button while you undo his pants, pull down his boxers, and begin sucking on his penis. Remember, you have to move fast, so make it a quick blow job (or a fast finger on the clitoris) in order to get off before anyone else needs to get on!

Hot and spicy: Stimulate yourself in the lady's room before heading to the elevator (or apply lubrication beforehand) so you're ready for quick entry once your lover gets on the elevator. As soon as the doors close, stimulate him by groping his crotch, unzipping his pants and pulling down his boxers, and fondling or sucking his penis. The goal is to get him hard as fast as possible. Once he's ready, lean against the wall, put a leg up on the railing, and let him thrust away.

Up the Ante

- Try a game of "Ride and Tease." The goal is not to orgasm, but to tease each other between floors so that you can have hot and steamy intercourse soon after. Start by getting on the elevator together. Push the button for every single floor and stand at the back. If no one gets on, kiss, fondle, and touch each other as much as possible before the elevator stops and the doors open. If other people are in front of you, discreetly fondle his crotch or let him grab your behind until you're alone again. As the doors open and close, continue this teasing action to build the excitement. Once you reach the top floor, repeat the game on the way down. Better yet, find a hidden stairwell, put one leg up on the railing, and let him enter you standing up to release the pent-up tension!

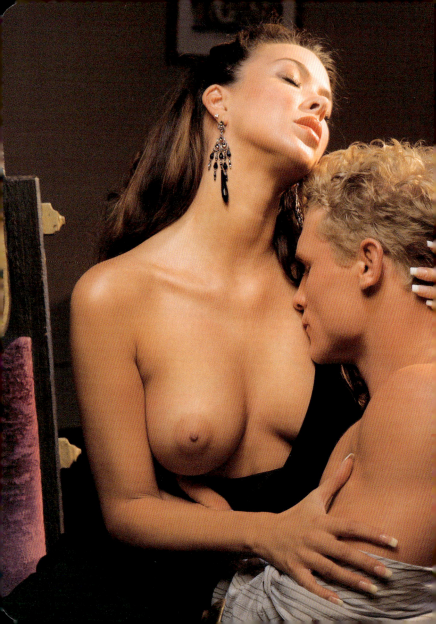

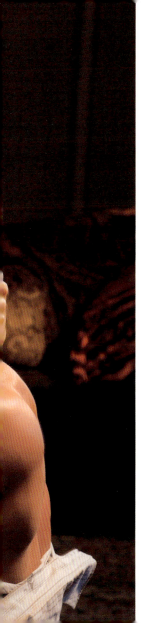

48

Ridin' the Rails

This is a great game to play if you're really traveling on a train (and can't wait for the sleeping car) or you're looking for a sexy adventure late at night.

The Sexy Setup

If your lover likes surprises, you can spring this game on her without any warning. If you know that she doesn't like surprises, tell her the two of you are going for a ride that involves pulling your engine in and out of her station.

Rules & Tools

After buying your ticket and selecting your seats, tell your lover you need to find the bathroom. Then check out the train and scout out an area for having sex, getting a quick blow job, or just opening her blouse, fondling her breasts, and sucking her nipples. Look for deserted cars, closets for stashing luggage, bathrooms, and the like.

Playing the Game

Sweet and safe: Stay right in your seats, but place one of your coats or a blanket over the two of you. Ask her to pull down her pants or pull up her skirt. Lubricate your fingers and start to stimulate her genitals.

Give her a circular clitoral orgasm: Run your first and second fingers in a circular motion around her pubic area and labia, then slide a finger quickly over her clitoris. Repeat the action over and over, building tension, until the last touch on her clitoris brings her to orgasm.

Hot and spicy: Once she's wet (or you're done with the above-mentioned game), take her hand and lead her to the location you've scouted out. Have her lean against the wall, and then bring her legs up around your waist while you thrust away to the motion of the train. Keep it up until you blow your whistle!

Up the Ante

- Play the sweet and safe game at the amusement park—if you can't bring her to orgasm on just one ride through the tunnel of love, get back in line and ride again until she comes. Then scout out a darkened alley, a deserted trolley car, or an abandoned ride to have her return the favor on you.

- Try any of these games in a moving Greyhound bus.

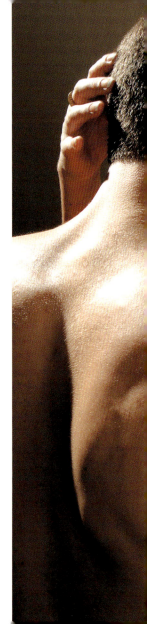

49

Restroom Rendezvous

Off to the museum, watching a ball game, or stuck at a conference all day? What better place for some quick and exciting sex than the local restroom?

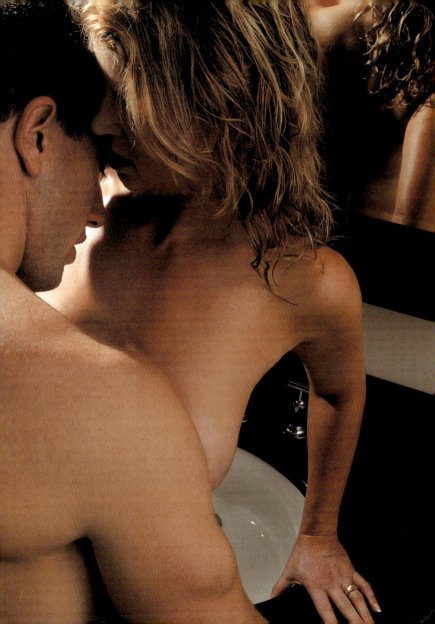

The Sexy Setup

If you and your lover are attending a conference, but listening to different sessions, send him a text message telling him you have something burning hot to talk to him about. Wandering through the museum together? Lean into him suggestively, letting your breast rub against his upper arm, and tell him to meet you in the last stall of the women's room at a certain time.

Rules & Tools

Time is of the essence with this game, so get yourself stimulated before your lover appears. Remember, if anyone looks under the door to see whether the stall is occupied, only one pair of shoes can show—preferably those of the appropriate sex!

Playing the Game

Sweet and safe: In the women's room: Have your lover stand on the toilet seat and let his pants slide off, presenting his penis right at your mouth level. Run your tongue up his thighs, fondle his buttocks, and cup his testicles in your hands. Once he's rock hard, give him a blow job or bring him to orgasm by hand, but be sure to catch his come in your mouth or a handful of tissue paper before you flush.

Hot and spicy: In the men's room: Remove your underclothes, then stand on the toilet seat, but raise one foot up onto the toilet paper holder to give him full access to your genitals. Hold the top of the stall or put your hands on the ceiling for extra support. Have your lover explore your thighs, labia, and clitoris with his tongue or insert a few fingers into your vagina or anus. Remember to keep your moans to a minimum if he brings you to orgasm.

Up the Ante

- Try having sex in a porta potty or in the restroom at a bar, a club, a restaurant, or an airport.

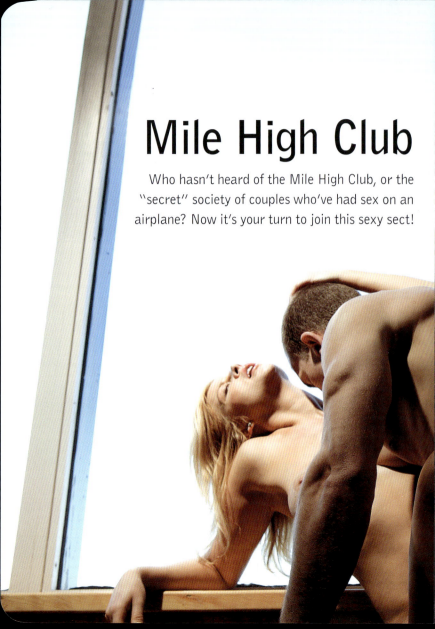

Mile High Club

Who hasn't heard of the Mile High Club, or the "secret" society of couples who've had sex on an airplane? Now it's your turn to join this sexy sect!

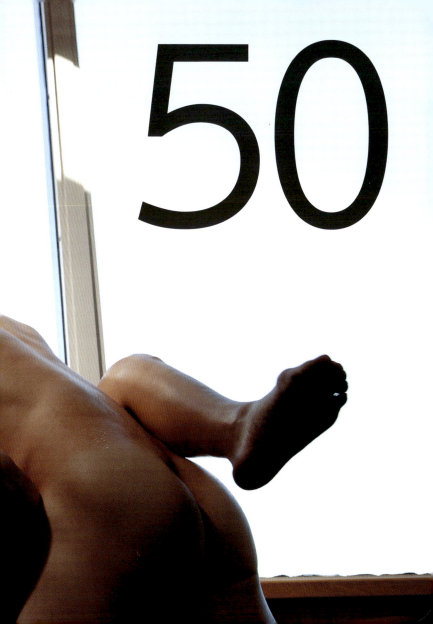

50

The Sexy Setup

This is a good game for surprising your lover, but if she doesn't like surprises you can start this game right in your seat, either by whispering suggestive ideas into her ear or fondling her thighs under the blanket.

Rules & Tools

You can try this game on just about any flight, but a red-eye flight (where the plane is flying overnight) is often the best choice, because most of the other passengers will be sleeping. If you get caught in the restroom, tell the other passengers or the flight attendant that your partner got sick and you were helping her out.

Playing the Game

Sweet and safe: Use this game as foreplay for meeting in the restroom, or bring each other to orgasm without leaving your seats. You'll need a blanket for covering your genitals. Start by kissing your lover's neck, then fondle her breasts. Ask her to slip off her panties and spread her legs so you can finger her to orgasm. To reciprocate, ask her to go down on you with the blanket over her head.

Hot and spicy: Head to the restroom separately. Work out a special knock so you can let her in once she arrives. There are plenty of different positions to try out, so this is a game that you can play over and over. Have your lover lean against the sink so you can enter her doggie style, sit on the sink and wrap her legs around your waist, or put one foot up on the toilet and enter her from behind. Prefer a seated position? Put the toilet seat down and sit on the seat, then have her climb on top facing the door. Fondle her breasts and hold on tight in case of unexpected turbulence!

Up the Ante

- Once you get home, play the "Flirty Flight Attendant" role-play game in chapter 6 (page 258).

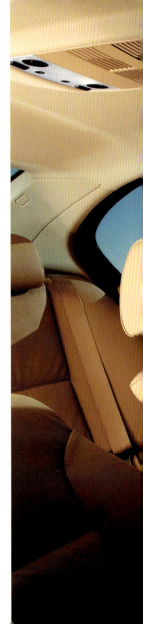

51

Auto-Erotica

Do you remember the days of making out in the backseat of your car? There's no reason you can't go back in time to play this updated version of Auto-Erotica!

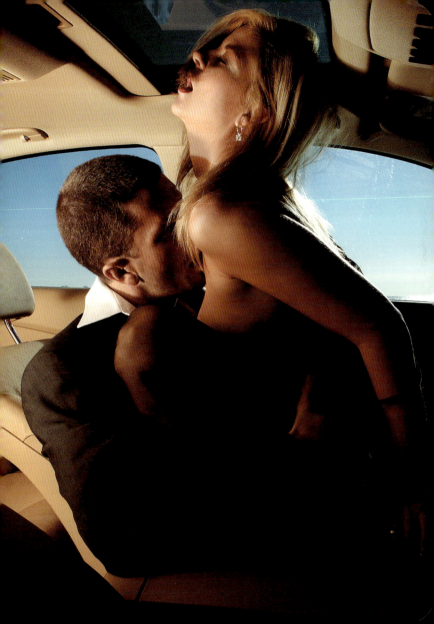

The Sexy Setup

Send your lover a note and tell him you're in need of a ride home. Take off all your clothes, but wear a long trench coat or raincoat to cover you up.

Rules & Tools

Stimulating your lover while he's driving is okay, but actually bringing him to orgasm while he's operating the vehicle could be dangerous. Far better to find a place to pull over and have sex in the car, on the hood, or even in the back of a pickup truck on a hot summer night.

Playing the Game

Sweet and safe: Start the game by flashing a little leg, breast, or belly while your lover is driving. Alternatively, begin touching yourself and moaning gently while he's operating the vehicle. Guaranteed he won't be able to keep his eyes on the road, so ask him to find a darkened parking lot or a deserted road. Once you're there, remove his pants, recline and push the driver's seat as far back as it goes, and jump on top of him (with the steering wheel at your back).

Hot and spicy: Give your lover a blow job while you're going through the car wash. If he doesn't come before the wash is over, keep fondling him while you drive somewhere remote. Once you're there, push the front seats as far forward as they go, ask him to lie down on the backseat, and ride him like a cowgirl!

Up the Ante

- Have your lover kneel with one leg on each front seat and push his penis toward you over the armrest. You sit in the backseat and suck him off.

- Get out of the car, lean over on the hood, and ask your lover to penetrate you from behind.

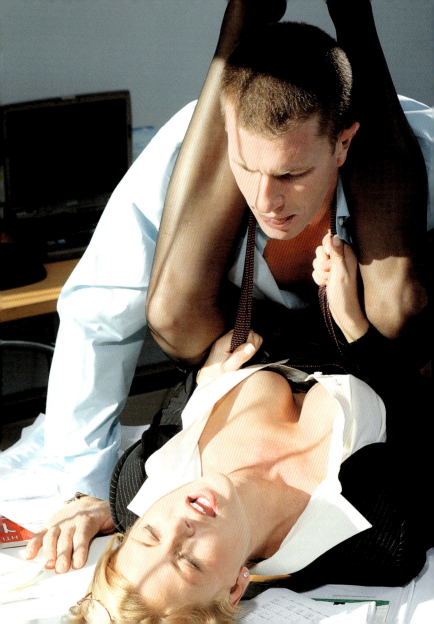

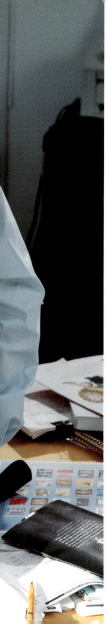

52

Hold My Calls
(and My Balls!)

Sometimes a man just can't wait till he gets home for a taste of his lover. There's no need to wait all day with this naughty office game!

The Sexy Setup

Call your lover and ask her if she's got a few minutes for a quick lunch or if you can meet her at her office after hours. Set a time you're going to meet, and mention that you're bringing a friend (use your favorite pet name for your penis).

Rules & Tools

If this is a daytime encounter, make sure you've scoped out her office ahead of time for empty closets, dead-end stairwells, offices that lock, or unused conference rooms. Bring along lubrication and plan a time when most people are out of the office, such as lunchtime or during a special meeting.

Playing the Game

Sweet and safe: Greet your lover with a passionate kiss, then lead her to the dead-end stairwell. Open her blouse and kiss, fondle, and tease her breasts, neck, and shoulders until she's wet, then lean her against the wall and enter her from behind or prop her on the stair railing and have her wrap her legs around your waist.

Hot and spicy: Tell her you'd really like to see her office. Once you're in, quickly close the door and lock it. Kiss her passionately while reaching under her skirt and pulling her panties down. Back her slowly up to her desk, clear off any critical papers, and lift her up onto the desk. Spread her legs and enter her standing up, with her vagina right at the edge of the desk, or lay her down and squeeze her nipples while you thrust away.

Up the Ante

- To up the thrill factor, seek out semiprivate areas for hot and steamy sex: a darkened corner of the corporate library, under the conference room table, or in the utility or coat closet. You can even lift her onto a copy machine, lay her on a lunchroom table, or do her on the waiting room couch!

- To heighten the excitement, add in a boss/secretary role-playing game.

53

Frisky Fun in the Furniture Store

A typical furniture store has many more beds, couches, and living room chairs than customers, making it the perfect forbidden spot for afternoon nooky!

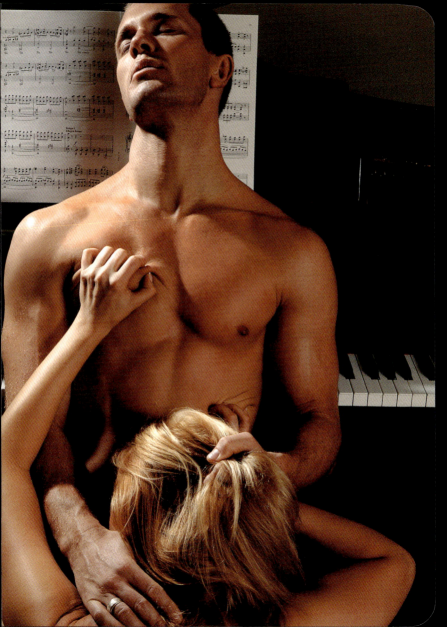

The Sexy Setup

Send your lover a note and tell him you'd like to go furniture shopping. Wear clothing that's easily removable, or be daring and wear a trench coat with nothing under it.

Rules & Tools

Take a long, meandering walk around the furniture store, scoping out spots that are off the beaten track or hard to get to. If there's a salesman lurking, be sure to tell him you prefer to shop alone.

Playing the Game

Sweet and safe: Find the most remote bed you can, take off your trench coat, lie down, and ask your lover to touch you all over. Once you're hot and wet, pull him onto you for a fast and furious furniture store quickie.

Hot and spicy: To play this game of cat and mouse, kiss your lover passionately in one location, then walk away. The next time he comes close, fondle his penis or buttocks through his clothes, but then move away. Flash him as you move through the store, or stop, sit in a chair, and start to masturbate. Don't stay put too long, however—as soon as he comes over, get up and move on to the next room. Continue this game until you're both hot, wet, and ready for sex. Find a comfortable bed or couch and get it on!

Up the Ante

- Play a game of "Test the Cushions." Once you're hot and wet, try having sex on as many cushions as possible. That means try all the beds, including the bunk beds, as well as the couches, chairs, recliners, and lounge chairs.

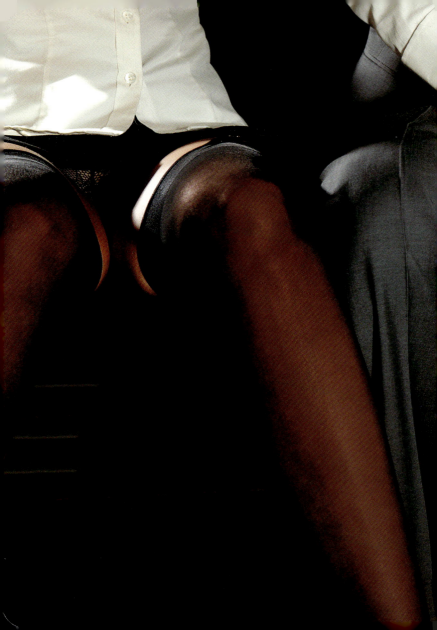

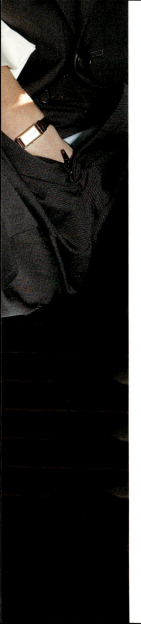

54

Movie Theater Hand Games

Remember the days of making out in the darkened movie theater? This adults-only version of the game is riskier, but the rewards are greater!

The Sexy Setup

Ask your lover on a date, and tell him you're headed for the movie theater. Mention that there may be some times when the off-screen action is hotter than expected!

Rules & Tools

The less populated the movie theater, the better (unless you really enjoy the thrill of possibly getting caught). Try going to an 11 a.m. showing time, or to a film that's been out for a while. Scout out the darkest corner of the theater, or the most remote seats. This game works best with a movie that contains a lot of action (the other viewers won't notice what's going on in the back corner) or one with a very loud soundtrack (to cover up your moans of pleasure!).

Playing the Game

Sweet and safe: Think of this game as pure foreplay, with the sex or orgasm destined to take place once you're back in the car or safely at home. As the movie begins, gently lean your breast against his upper arm, slide your hand onto his thigh, and lean over to kiss his neck.

As the movie action builds, begin fondling his penis from the outside of his pants until he's hard. If necessary, put your coat over his lap to cover the action. As the movie gets louder, undo his pants and slip your hand inside. Stroke, fondle, and rub his penis, testicles, or groin area, but try not to bring him to orgasm. Instead, leave him hard, which will keep him revved up for sex later on!

Hot and spicy: Wear a skirt with no undergarments, and bring along lubrication or your favorite miniature vibrator. Tell your lover you're so horny you can't wait until you get home, so you want him to get you off during the movie. Place a coat over your lap to cover the action, then lube up his fingers or hand him the vibrator. Spread your legs, close your eyes, and let your lover's hands bring you to the edge of your seat!

Up the Ante

- Once you're hot and horny from the sweet and safe game and the film is over, find a hidden corner, slip into an unused restroom, or proceed toward a little-used exit and let him penetrate you standing up, leaning over, or even on the floor.

55

Let's Hear That Engine Purr

Men love their toys, especially those with engines. The next time you need a naughty tryst, try mounting him while seated on a motorcycle or ride-on lawn mower!

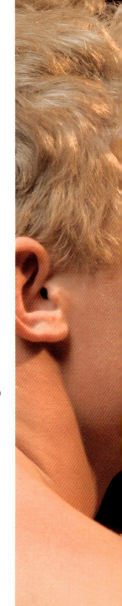

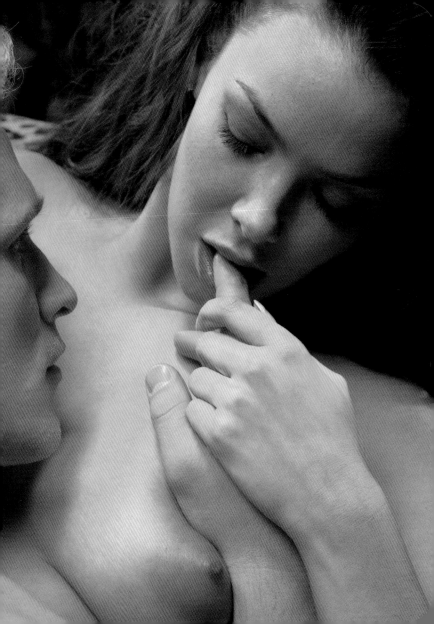

The Sexy Setup

Tell your lover to meet you in the garage or toolshed. Put on your sexiest lingerie (it will contrast beautifully with the dirty tools and motor grease) under a trench coat or bathrobe and tell him you want to hear his engine hum.

Rules & Tools

If the garage or toolshed is unheated, consider bringing a blanket or two for post-coital cuddling. Move any sharp tools or garden implements out of the way, and take care if you're walking barefoot or moving around unclothed. If you plan to run the motorcycle or lawn mower, be sure to open a window for ventilation.

Playing the Game

Sweet and safe: Sit on the bike and slip off your coat or robe to reveal your lingerie. Tell him you're trying out for a pinup calendar like the ones you find in garages, then strike a few suggestive poses while sitting on the bike. Lie down with your feet on the handlebars, rub your genitals against the bike seat, and strike as many provocative poses as possible while he watches. Once you're both hot and wet, have sex doggie style over the bike's saddle.

Hot and spicy: Sit on the bike together, either facing each other (for lap sex) or leaning away from him (for rear entry). Ask him to start the engine but put on the safety break. Have sex in time to the vibrations of the motorcycle.

Up the Ante

- Undress your lover using your sexiest moves, then stimulate him with your hands or mouth to get him hard. Ask him to sit on the seat of his ride-on lawn mower and start the engine. Climb on top of him, facing him for one game or facing away (as if you're driving the mower) for another. Let the mower's vibrating engine add to the sensation of ride-on sex!

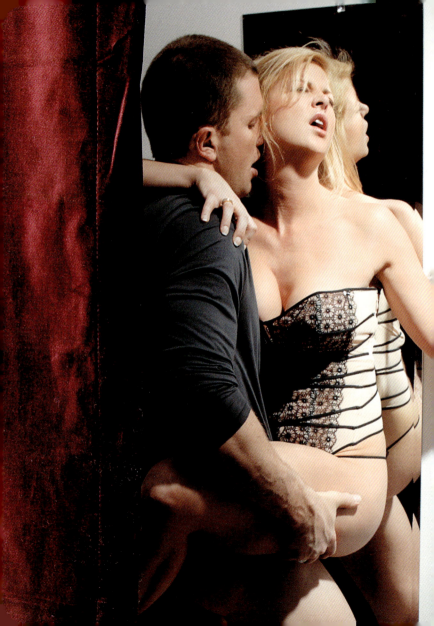

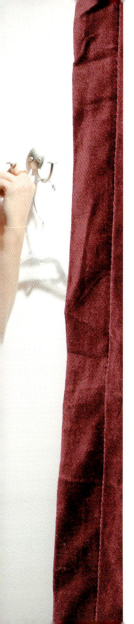

56

The Un-Dressing Room

This is a game that's fun for both parties—
you get some new clothes and some sexual
satisfaction in the same day!

The Sexy Setup

Tell your lover you'd like to go shopping, but you need him to rate your outfits. Mention that you're planning to model a number of different ensembles, from full-length gowns to lingerie and bathing suits.

Rules & Tools

Scout out the stores ahead of time to locate the least-visited or most private dressing rooms. Plan to visit the store when it's not too busy, such as in the evening, an hour before closing, or other off hours. (Of course, if you're feeling really daring you can try this game on a weekend afternoon, a national day off from work, or right around the holidays when the stores tend to be busiest!)

Playing the Game

Sweet and safe: Stroll around the store together, arm in arm, looking at clothing, lingerie, dresses, and even shoes and hats. Ask him what colors and fabrics he likes, or what style of things he'd like to see you model. If possible, really reach outside your comfort zone and pick out some sexy, suggestive, or even slutty clothing. The hotter the better!

Take the clothing back to the dressing room, and find him a seat just outside the dressing room. One by one, model the outfits, taking your time to turn slowly, flash him some leg or breast, or just come close to him. Make sure you ask him which outfit he likes the best, and buy that one for additional fun later on!

Hot and spicy: If your sweet and safe game is really turning him on, invite him into the dressing room. Ask him to help you put on his favorite outfit by zipping you in or fastening your buttons. As his fingers do the work, ask him to stop at certain places and explore. Give him a couple of hot, passionate kisses and some gentle groping to get him hard, then slip off the garments and have sex against the wall, on the dressing room floor, or even on the little seat. Use the mirror for added stimulation!

Up the Ante

- Wear your sexy outfit over to the men's dressing rooms. Make sure you flash a few of the other men or flirt with your eyes; your lover will enjoy knowing he's got you all to himself while surrounded by other men.

57

Sex in Space

Believe it or not, scientists have spent considerable time researching how to have sex without gravity. There's no need to wait for the space station, however— you can play with your space needle right at home!

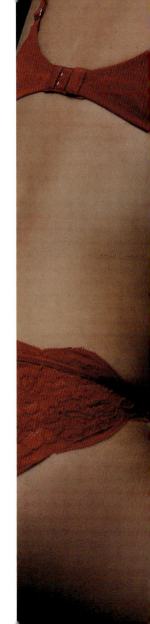

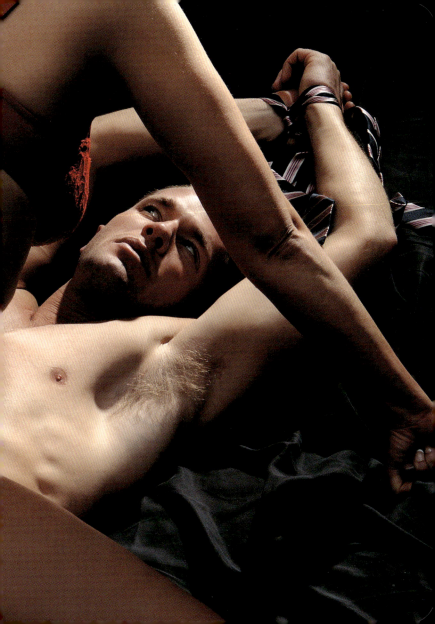

The Sexy Setup

Invite your lover over for a game of *Lost in Space, Star Trek*, or *Star Wars*. Pick your favorite female character and assign him the male version. Then tell him you're going to be the first humans to have sex with no gravity.

Rules & Tools

The key is to pretend you're in outer space and there's no gravity. What, exactly, does that mean? You'll need to stay anchored down—with ties, belts, scarves or whatever you can find. And you can have fun making any liquids that you use (or produce) "fly" all around too.

Playing the Game

Sweet and safe: Keeping two bodies together in zero-G will be difficult, if not impossible, so one partner has to be anchored to the bed, couch, or floor. Use whatever you have on hand—ties, belts, or silk scarves—to keep your partner from floating away as you prepare to lick him from head to toe. Remember to hold on to him every second, however, to prevent yourself from floating away!

Hot and spicy: Scientists say men may experience a slight decrease in penis size while having sex in space. This is because humans in microgravity typically have lower blood pressure. To counter that, you're going to work extra hard to keep him extra hard, whether that means biting gently along his inner thighs, gently sucking his testicles, or stimulating him with two hands. Remember, any lubrication might just float off into space, so the more you can use your mouth to keep him hard, the better!

Up the Ante

- Fashion some space-age bondage for counteracting the loss of gravity. Outfit you and your partner with several straps made of Velcro. Once you're in position for having sex, the Velcro will prevent you from floating away.

- Tie one of each of your hands to the bed to counter the effects of zero-G and try kissing, stimulating each other, or having sex with just one hand.

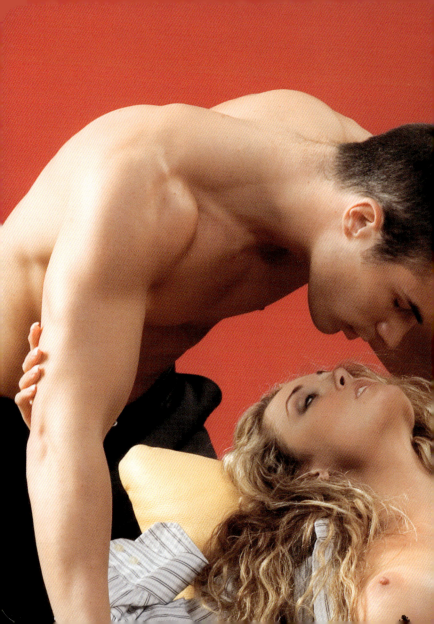

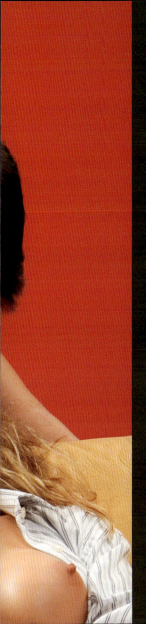

CHAPTER 6

What's Your Fantasy?

Who among us doesn't like to pretend we're someone else once in a while, and when you add sex and naughtiness to that scenario, you have some fun role-playing games that are sure to spice things up- and keep it hot for months to come! (With all role-playing games, you and your lover should agree ahead of time on a safe word, or a word that when spoken means "stop.")

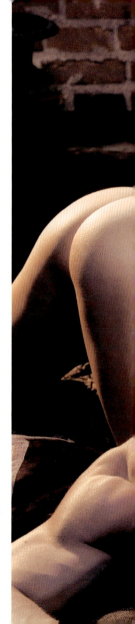

58

Door-to-Door Vibrator Salesman

This fantasy game is purrrrrfect for men who like to role-play . . . and pull out all the toys!

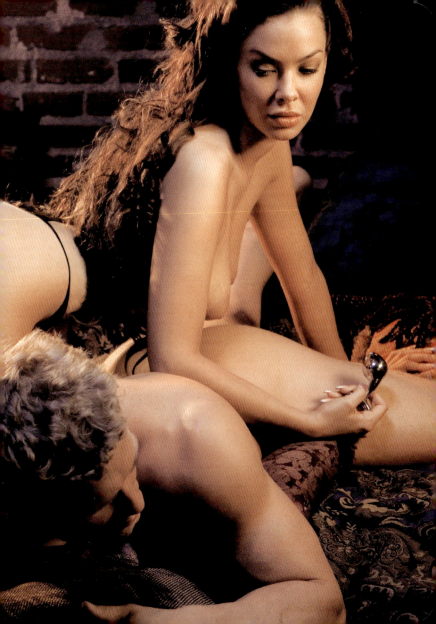

The Sexy Setup

Here's the game: You're going to dress in a suit and arrive at your home, pretending to be a door-to-door vibrator salesman. To pull this off, you've got to try and surprise your lover when she thinks you're off at work (or busy doing something else). Alternatively, tell her you're going out for a while, then ring the doorbell a few minutes later and start the game!

Rules & Tools

Wear a suit and carry a briefcase with pamphlets and a selection of vibrators. For the hot and spicy version of the game, be sure your briefcase is complete with ties and handcuffs.

Playing the Game

Sweet and safe: Ring the doorbell, then come into the house and explain that you have some very exciting products to show her. Take out the vibrators one by one, taking your time handling each one and explaining which are best suited for what types of play. Ask her if she'd like to borrow one and try it out (with you watching, of course!).

Hot and spicy: Come into the house and lay down the rules: You can only show her the products if she's naked, so the first thing she has to do is strip down (or get into something comfortable, like a short and sexy bathrobe). What's more, you're going to demonstrate their effectiveness on her whether she likes it or not. At this point you can pull out some silk ties or handcuffs and bind her arms or legs to a chair leg. Then run through the product line one by one, taking as much time as you like to demonstrate just how effective the devices are for stimulation, teasing, and perhaps even orgasm.

Up the Ante

- Ask her swap roles and test the vibrators on you—perhaps you'd like to try anal stimulation!

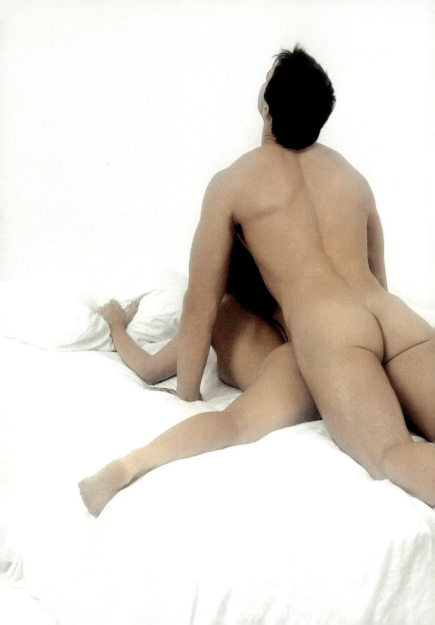

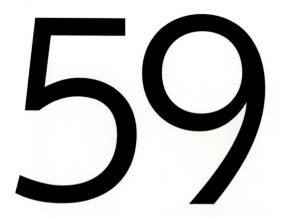

59

Under House Arrest

This sexy game of dominance and submission gives new meaning to the phrase "frisk me." And what man can resist playing policeman for a night?

The Sexy Setup

Tell your lover you want to play cops and robbers. You're going to represent the law, and she's going to be the bad girl who just got caught shoplifting.

Rules & Tools

Wear a pair of dark sunglasses and bring along a pair of handcuffs.

Playing the Game

Sweet and safe: Take control of this game: You've nabbed her committing a crime, and now it's time for you to check her out. Have her stand and face the wall, arms up and open. Pat her down all over, taking your time on her breasts, belly, or bottom. At the end cuff her, then turn her around and order her to suck you off—or else.

Hot and spicy: Start with a little game of chase around the house (but make sure you catch her!). Tell her you're going to perform a strip search, then take your time checking out all her crevices. Once the strip search is done, order her to get down on the floor, facedown, legs and arms spread-eagle. Frisk her from this position, but let your hands go (and stay!) wherever they want, because you're the law. Once she's hot and wet, spread her legs and enter her from behind. Be sure to pin her hands down so she can't move.

Up the Ante

• Use the element of surprise to your advantage—
  in other words, she doesn't know when this game's
  going to happen! Sneak into the house when she
  thinks you've gone somewhere else. Your aim:
  to surprise and/or scare her—the adrenaline rush
  she'll get from being scared can quickly turn to lust.
  (Just make sure she doesn't call 911 or you'll both be
  in hot water!)

60

Flirty Flight Attendant

This is a good game for women who like to be dominant and men who like taking orders from a woman in charge!

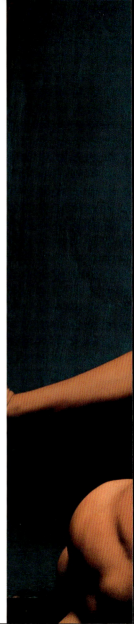

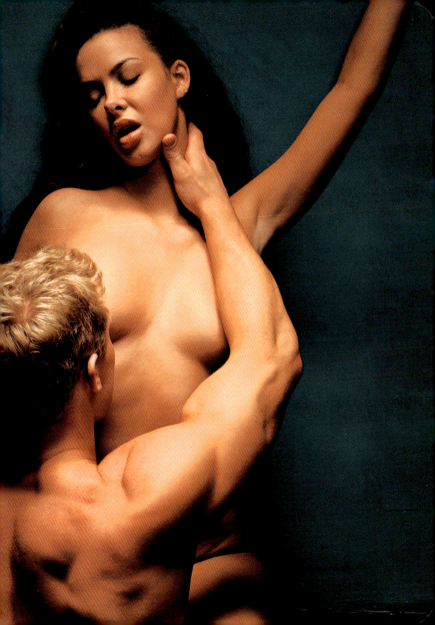

The Sexy Setup

Tell your lover you have a naughty game where he's the passenger and you're the flirty flight attendant who's going to teach him a lesson about proper in-flight conduct.

Rules & Tools

Set up the scene beforehand. Dress in your sexiest flight attendant outfit, complete with stockings, heels, and lingerie. Have some props on hand, such as a drink tray, cups, peanuts, and napkins, as well as a small pillow, a blanket, an eye cover (the kind they give out on overnight flights), and a pair of handcuffs. Next, find a chair in your house that resembles an airline seat and prepare for take-off!

Playing the Game

Sweet and safe: Have your lover play airplane traveler by asking for food or drinks, but then do things by "accident" to upset you. He can spill his drink, ask for multiple pillows, etc. When you get annoyed, have him try to kiss you or touch you inappropriately (and keep trying). Once you're completely fed up, tell him you're going to restrain him—then pull out a pair of cuffs and fasten his hands behind him.

Now it's your turn to take the game wherever you want by teasing him with a flash of your breasts, man-handling him until he's hard, or demanding he follow your every command and satisfy you *now*!

Hot and spicy: Follow the same game as above, but step it up a notch on the bossy (or bitchy) scale. When he spills his drink, lean across him in a bossy manner and accidentally bump your breasts into his face; if he tries to kiss you, push him around or slap him gently. When he asks for more drinks or pillows, alternate between acting put out and being ready to put out. Remove your stockings in a teasing manner, making sure he gets a good view of your thighs and genitals, and then use the stockings to tie him to the chair. Begin your punishment by undressing him from the waist down, then teasing him using your hands, mouth, and lips. Each time he seems ready to orgasm, pull away. Once you're hot and wet, climb on him and take him to new heights of passion!

Up the Ante

- Before you restrain him, get into a gentle struggle (but let him win). Have him tie you to the chair, then either tease you into submission or take you forcibly while you fight back.

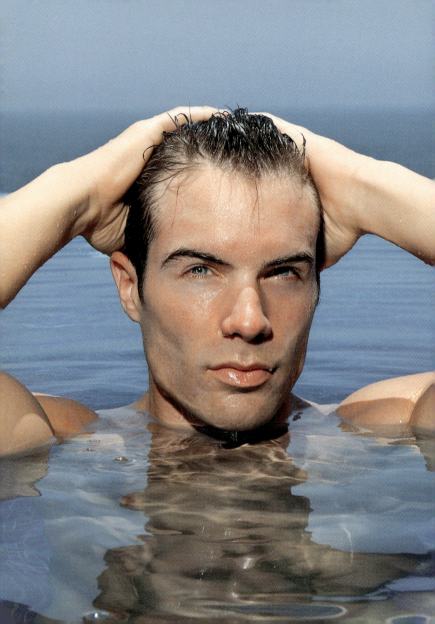

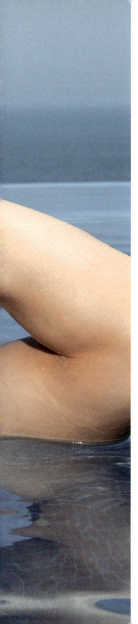

61

Handyman Come Calling

This is every stay-at-home mom's fantasy: the hot and randy handyman who's handy in more ways than one!

The Sexy Setup

Tell your lover you have a secret game for her, but you're not going to tell her what it is until the game begins. She should just be home alone when you come knocking!

Rules & Tools

Dress the part—put on a pair of dirty jeans, work boots, and a big sweatshirt or heavy jacket. Borrow a tool belt and load it up with sex toys, lubricant, or silk ties, but keep it under your jacket so she doesn't see it at first. (Alternatively, bring along the same items in a bucket or shop bag.)

Playing the Game

Sweet and safe: Ring the doorbell, and when she answers, tell her you're the handyman whose come to help around the house. Ask her what needs fixing—are her drawers squeaky? Do the bedsprings need attention? Depending on her answer, lead her to the room where you can best play the game, then tell her you're handy in more ways than one. Ask her where your hands are most needed: To undress her slowly? To caress her breasts and nipples? To stimulate her clitoris? Then get to work!

Hot and spicy: Ring the doorbell, introduce yourself, and take charge. Lead her from room to room, slowly building the seduction and asking her what she needs fixed. Offer to change the lightbulb, but brush up against her suggestively; kiss her ankles as you pretend to look under the couch, or grab her from behind as she moves from room to room. Once you've settled on a room, take off your coat and show her your tools, then tell her you're especially handy with tools that penetrate, applying lubricant where it's most needed, and screwing things in. Demonstrate just how handy you are until she's hot and wet, then strip down and *nail her* on the floor.

Up the Ante

- Surprise your lover by wearing a tool belt—and nothing else. Make yourself hard before you walk in the room and she's sure to melt at the sight of your biggest tool!

62

Horny Housemaid

Here's a great game for the man
who likes to be serviced—and a woman
who likes to take care of her man.

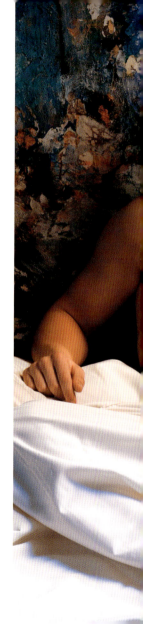

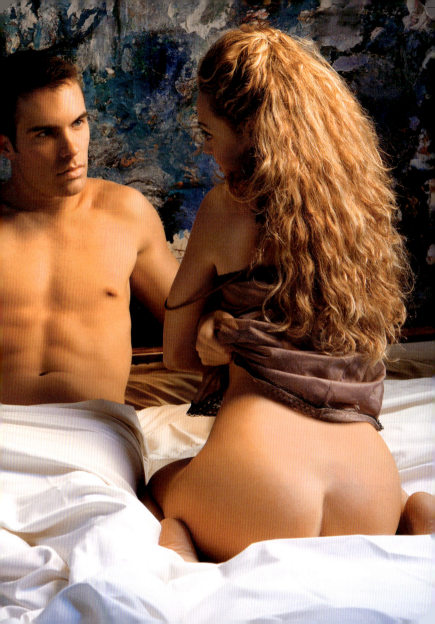

see if he's watching you. There are two options: Really draw out the submissive act, moving suggestively around the room, then suddenly strip off the housedress, shake out your hair, and pounce on him. Or remove the outfit piece by piece in a seductive striptease, emerging at the end as a tempting temptress ready to clean his house!

ames Bible

Hot and spicy: Pretend he's the overworked, lonesome bachelor who's relaxing with his favorite drink—and getting ready to watch an adult film. Knock on the door and call out, "Maid service, may I come in?" Start tidying up the room, making sure you lean over suggestively, flashing him a peak under your skirt. Sit next to him and ask if there's anything that needs special attention—after all, you're at his service and you aim to please. Perhaps he needs help undressing so you can do the laundry, or would he like you to turn on the movie for him? Take off his clothes and leave the room, then come back suddenly (and catch him masturbating). Tell him that's your job, and take over with your hands, mouth, and lips. Make sure you clean up any extra mess you make!

Up the Ante

- Play a game of "Masturbating Maid." Tie him up with your apron and tease or tickle him with your feather duster. Once he's tied up, slowly undress yourself, stroking your nipples, caressing your breasts, and fingering your clitoris. Bring yourself to climax while he's tied down and forced to watch, then ask him how you can be of *service*!

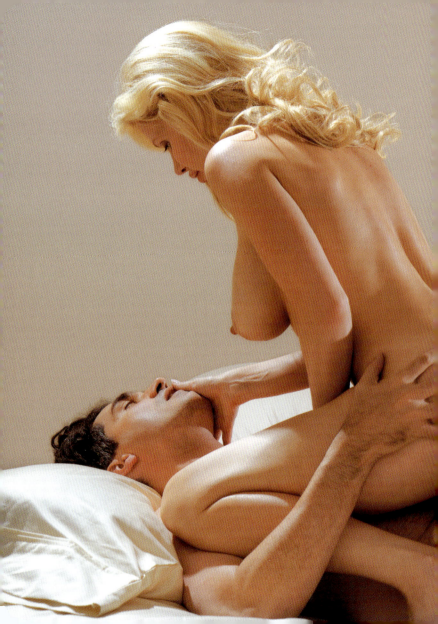

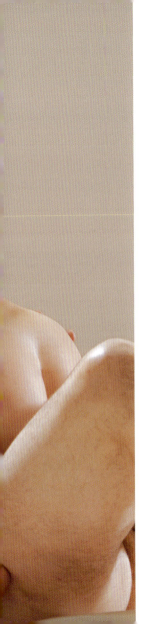

63

Visiting Nurse

Here's another game for the man who likes to be serviced—and the woman who enjoys teasing her lover while being dominant.

answers the door, announce that you're the visiting nurse come to follow up on his problem. When he asks what problem that is, tell him you received a lab report indicat-

Ask him to lie on the couch and remain motionless while you check him out. Undress him slowly and check out every inch of him, avoiding the genitals until he's squirming, all the while flashing him a peek of your lingerie or red bra. Get him hot, then massage his penis and bring him to orgasm. It's your job to make him feel better!

Hot and spicy: Step up the role-playing and act like a bossy nurse who's short on time (and patience). Strip off his clothes, then examine him a little roughly. Pull on the rubber gloves and examine his genitals in great detail, perhaps flicking your tongue over his balls or even probing his anus. Open your tool kit and use your tools or toys to probe and examine all your lover's body parts and crevices. Be sure to flash him a glimpse of your garter strap, your own genitals, or your sexy lingerie to heighten his response. Once he's hot and hard, climb on top and ride him to orgasm—this visiting nurse is all business!

Up the Ante

- Cook up a different scenario: Your husband is at a fertility clinic to donate sperm. He's alone in the donation room with his raunchy magazines and a cup, and you (the nurse) accidentally open the door!

64

Pirate and Captive Maiden

You can play your own version of Captain Jack Sparrow with this role-playing game—just get ready to capture the bootie!

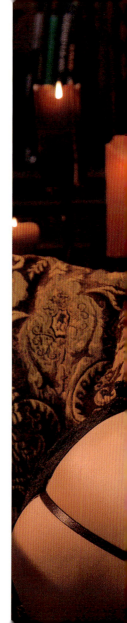

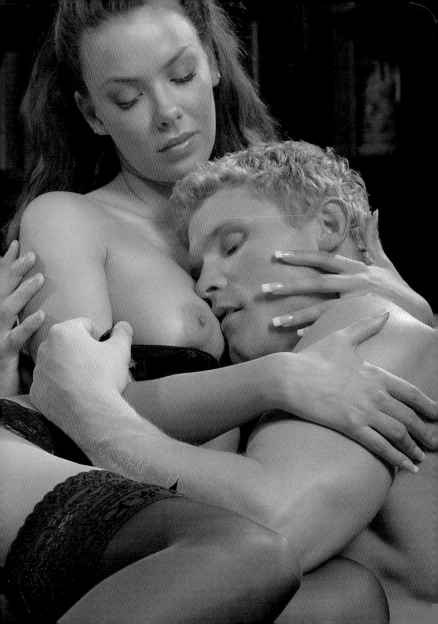

The Sexy Setup

Tell your lover you have a swashbuckling game in mind:
You're going to be the pirate and she gets to play the captive maiden. If she's willing, ask her to dress in a maiden's
outfit, like a dress with a low-cut top, plenty of jewelry,
and a full skirt (with no undergarments!).

Rules & Tools

You need to dress like a pirate for this game, whether that
means buying a costume or making your own. Take your
inspiration from books and movies: Wrap your head in a
bandanna, darken your eyes, put on a big white shirt unbut-
toned to your waist, slip into your tightest pants, and put
on your seafaring boots. Collect your props, such as an eye
patch, a hook for a hand, or a toy parrot on your shoulder.

Playing the Game

Sweet and safe: Open the game with this line: "Ahoy,
mates! Keep your hands off the Captain's maiden!" Then
pretend you're protecting her from a room full of leering
faces and dozens of hands by pulling her onto your lap,
stroking her hair, and kissing her bosom.

Reach under her skirt and secretly pleasure her while the other pirates continue drinking, eating, and making noise. She's your captive, but you're her protector!

Hot and spicy: This time she's your captive, but you're the horny pirate who's been at sea far too long. It's been months since you've seen a woman, let alone touched one, and she's beautiful to boot. Tie her hands behind her back and manhandle her breasts, or rip off her dress and tie her naked to a chair for your viewing pleasure. Tease her breasts and nipples with your lips and mouth until she's wet, then pull her hair and kiss her roughly. Take her any way you want—you're the captain of this boat!

Up the Ante

- If your lover is willing, make her your sex slave. Rip her clothes off, then make her perform all the duties of a captive maiden completely naked. That might include hoisting the sails (removing your clothing), walking the beam (sucking you off), and swabbing the deck (cleaning up the mess!).

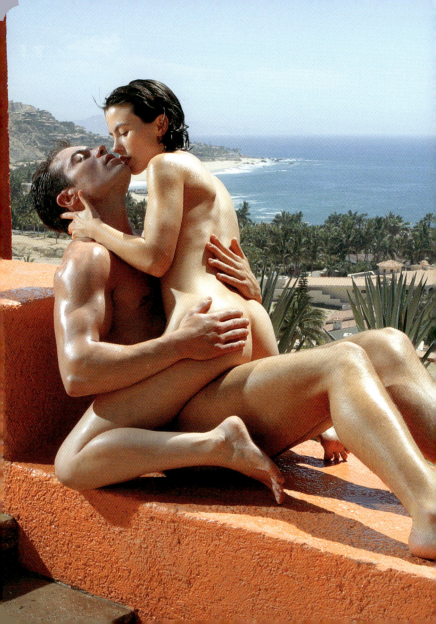

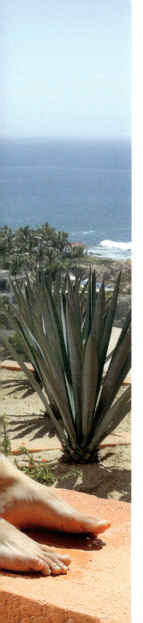

65

Mistress
(or Master) and
Sex Slave

Do you love the idea of having your own personal sex slave? Do you tingle at the thought of ordering your lover to pleasure you whenever you want? Then this is the game for you.

The Sexy Setup

Tell your lover that you have a game he's sure to love (especially if he likes being dominated). Tell him you're the beautiful princess, and he's the handsome sex slave who must do (or wear) whatever his mistress desires.

Rules & Tools

Dress in your favorite princess outfit: Put on your sexiest bikini-style top, bikini bottoms (preferably with an attached loincloth), and decorative belt, choker, and armbands. Dress your lover in a loincloth or nothing at all. Assemble a pair of handcuffs, choker, or other props as desired.

Playing the Game

Sweet and safe: Order your lover to give you pleasure, whether that means feeding you by hand, massaging your feet, or brushing your hair. If you want him to caress your breasts, suck your nipples, or squeeze your butt, order him to do so until you want him to stop. Direct him to all your favorite spots, and order him to do whatever feels good for you. Remember, this is all about your pleasure—and as slave, he must do whatever his mistress wants.

Hot and spicy: Swap roles, and ask him to handcuff your hands together. Now you're his sex slave, and he's the master. He can order you to lick his entire body, let him penetrate you anally, or he can expose parts of you for his own pleasure—he's in control.

Up the Ante

• Buy your lover a choker and leash and lead him from room to room like a dog. When you want pleasure, tell him to do it (or face punishment). Keep a paddle or crop on hand for punishing his failure to pleasure you completely or showing any sign of disrespect.

• Take it outside: Make your lover go places in public without undergarments or masturbate in a public place (while you watch). Remember, you're in charge!

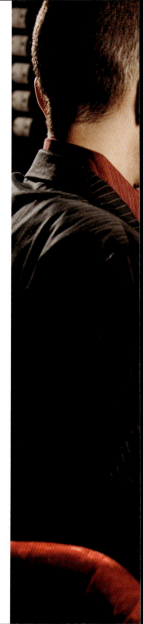

66

Pickup
at the Bar

Here's a fun game for spicing up your
relationship. This is especially well suited
for couples who need a pick-me-up in the
adventure department!

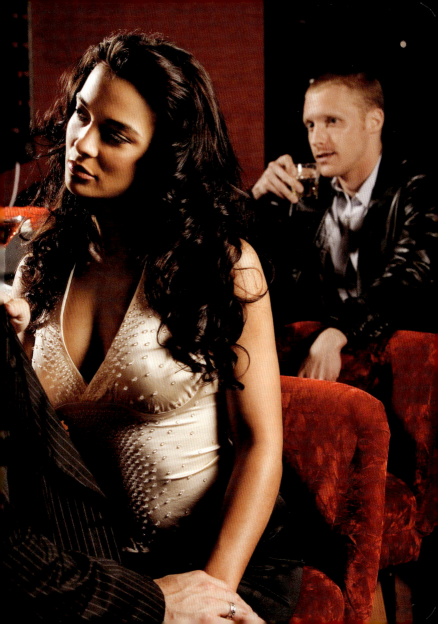

The Sexy Setup

Make a plan ahead of time with your lover, then send her a sexy note to remind her of the details. "Meet me at Oliver's at 8 p.m.; be sure to wear your sexiest outfit."

Rules & Tools

Decide ahead of time where you're heading after the pickup: back to your place, to a hotel room, to the car, etc. You should also decide who gets picked up and who is on the prowl (swap roles the next time) and whether flirting with other patrons is okay or off limits. But don't plan out the dialogue or the action—leave some room for spontaneity.

Playing the Game

Sweet and safe: Ask her to dress the part she wants to play—here's her chance to move outside her comfort zone. Maybe she's got a new top with a plunging neckline that you haven't seen, a short skirt that shows off her legs, or a pair of thigh-high boots that she's been dying to wear. Tell her to find a spot at the bar and let you do the work. She can play hard to get, act like a tease, or flirt openly. Draw out the pickup as long as possible to heighten the tension.

Hot and spicy: Add some role-playing to your game. Tell her to pretend she's been stood up and she's angry at men in general; this way, you'll have to seduce her by playing extra nice. Or have her act like a slut, tease you a bit, then take you by the hand and give you a steamy blow job in the men's bathroom or a hidden closet. Alternatively, act like a shy, geeky virgin who needs instruction from an experienced older woman.

Up the Ante

- Invite a female friend to join in (but don't tell your lover). Ask your friend to flirt with your lover openly—a little competition can add some spice to the situation (as long as things don't get out of hand). Have a secret word or code for when it's time to back off completely.

- Alternatively, invite a male friend to join in (but don't tell your lover). Have your friend flirt openly with your lover or even try and pick her up. Chances are his attention will boost her ego (and he may turn her on in different ways). Have a secret word for when it's time to back off completely so you can complete the pickup!

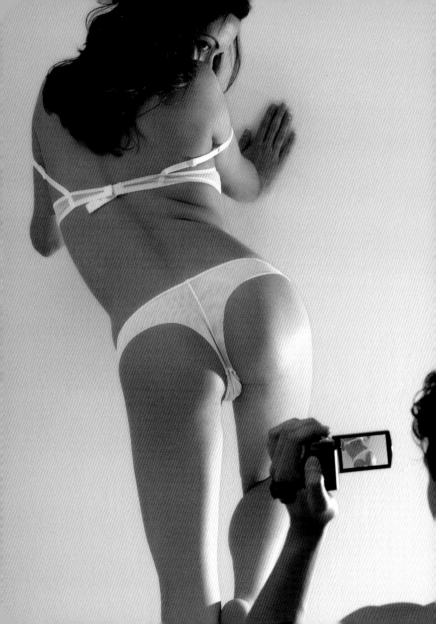

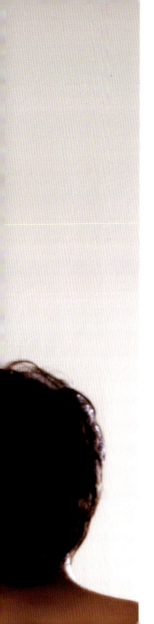

67

Porn Star and Director

This is a fun game for either sex—one gets to be the budding porn star (or centerfold model) while the other person plays director. Roll the cameras!

The Sexy Setup

Tell your lover you want her to play the budding centerfold and/or porn star, and you're the director of the photo shoot. As a virgin to the industry, she must follow your every command.

Rules & Tools

Set up a sexy area for her photo shoot, such as a fur-covered couch, a bed with silk sheets, or a bearskin rug in front of the fire. Keep different props and sex toys nearby (hot and spicy). Ask her to dress in her sexiest lingerie or bikini, but to wear a short robe over her outfit.

Load your camera with film (or charge your digital camera) and/or set up your camcorder or handheld video camera. Dress like this is all business. If you really want your photos to look authentic, buy a few porn magazines ahead of time and study the photos.

Playing the Game

Sweet and safe: Have your lover pose for her centerfold shots, but tell her it's all about looking sensuous and sexy. You can direct her to remove her clothing, fondle herself, lean over suggestively, lie on her stomach and expose her buttocks, or pull her lingerie aside to expose her genitals. Take photos of each pose, then organize them into a slideshow and watch it together.

Hot and spicy: Tell your lover this photo shoot is for a true porn magazine, and she has to do whatever turns you on (even if she objects)—pinch her own nipples, finger herself, or wear handcuffs so you can insert a butt plug or dildo (and then take pictures). Now's the time to pose her in the way you've always imagined her, or to ask her to act out *your* favorite fantasies!

Up the Ante

- Get out the camcorder or video camera and shoot a movie, such as *Naughty Nympho* or *I Can't Stop Masturbating*. Give your lover her lines, direct her moves, and film away!

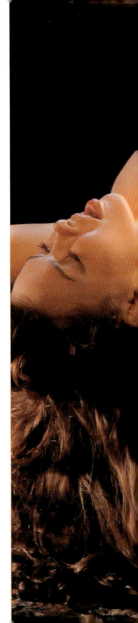

68

Surprise Sex

This is a fun game based on fear,
suspense—and pleasure, of course!

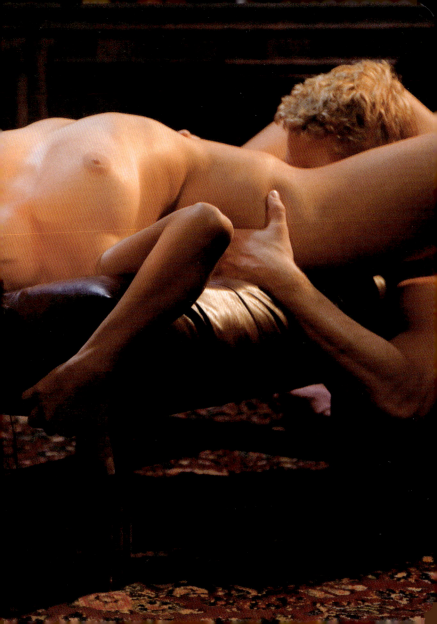

The Sexy Setup

Tell your lover you're going to play a game of surprise sex, and she's going to star in this game.

Rules & Tools

You'll need a bed or footstool, a blindfold, and lubrication. (You can also use sex toys if desired.)

Playing the Game

Sweet and safe: Slowly and sensuously undress your lover, and have her lie naked on the bed or footstool. Blindfold her, then lubricate different parts of your body, such as your fingers, knuckles, toes, elbows, chin, nose, genitals, and so on. Touch her in various places and ask her to guess which part of your body you're touching her with. Draw this out and have fun—try and caress her breasts with your toes, massage her clitoris with your knuckle, or rub her labia with your lubricated elbow.

Hot and spicy: Tell your lover to imagine the bed as a boat, you as a shark, and her as the victim. Pretend you're the shark, silently creeping up to attack the boat. Circle the bed or footstool while she tries to guess where you are. Build suspense by coming at the victim from various angles. Tickle her nipples, then suck her toes. Nibble her breasts with your teeth, or run a fingernail down the inside of her thigh. Stay clear of the genitals as you build suspense. Stop moving for a few minutes to heighten her anticipation, then suddenly kiss her hard and fondle her genitals. Move away again, then continue the teasing and suspense until she's quivering in anticipation. Finish the game however suits you best!

Up the Ante

- Use your favorite sex toys to tease or stimulate your partner, bring along a feather, or introduce other household items to build suspense.

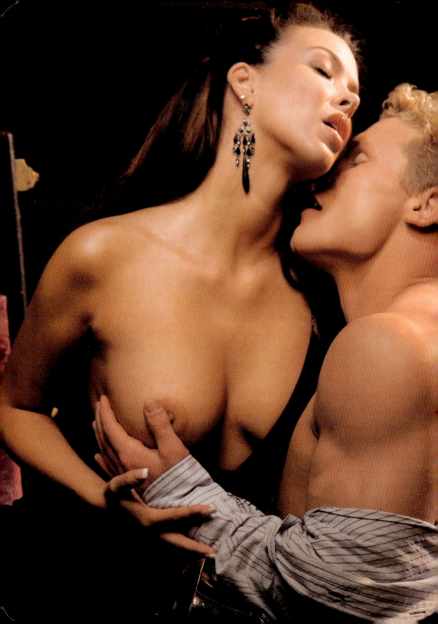

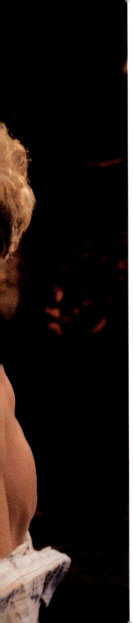

69

Hooker and Client

This is a game that can be played over and over in lots of different ways. You're selling your body, and he's the buyer.

The Sexy Setup

Tell your lover you need a ride home from work, a friend's house, a restaurant, etc. and you have a fantasy game you want to play. Arrange a date and time for him to pick you up. (You can pick up your car later.)

Rules & Tools

Dress the part of a call girl or hooker: Find your sexiest, sleaziest, or most daring outfit and put it on. Wear high heels, fishnet stockings, and plenty of makeup. (Wear a trench coat over your outfit if you need to be discreet.)

Playing the Game

Sweet and safe: When your lover arrives, ask him to roll down the window. Lean over, flashing him a good look at your cleavage, and ask him if he's looking for a little fun. (He should pick up on the game at this point, but if he doesn't, mention that you have a whole bag of tricks for sale.) Climb into the car and ask him what he'd like to buy—a quickie or a blow job—then tell him the price. Ask him to drive somewhere remote, and get down to business!

Hot and spicy: As you lean in the window, ask your lover what his wildest fantasy is. Name your price, and assuming he accepts, have him drive you to a prearranged spot (hotel room, home, etc.) where you can act out his fantasy. Remember, he's buying and you're performing the service, so it's all about pleasuring him!

Up the Ante

- Reverse the roles, and have him play the part of a male escort or gigolo. Have him dress in a tux or fancy clothes, then take him out on the town and parade him around. Once you get home, order him to perform whatever service you can afford!

70

Farm Girl in the Hay

Every man fantasizes about a romp in the clover with the lonely farm girl or a quickie in the hay with the milkmaid. Here's your chance to act out that fantasy in the privacy of your own home.

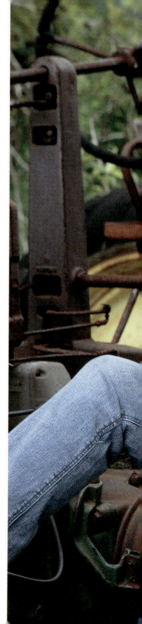

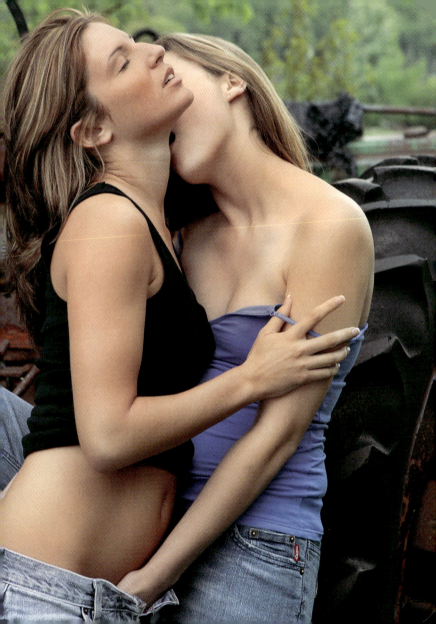

The Sexy Setup

Tell your lover you have a game to play, then describe one of the roles for you (and one for him) as detailed below.

Rules & Tools

Pick a role: the innocent virgin farm girl who needs sex instruction, the naughty milkmaid who likes nooky in the hay, or the quiet, shy girl next door who's really a vixen at heart. Arrange a date and time for him to come visit you, and give him a role to play: the experienced farmhand, the farmer's shy and timid son, or the horny teenager next door who masturbates every night.

Playing the Game

Sweet and safe: If you're the innocent virgin farm girl, dress in overalls, with a tiny top underneath. Put your hair in pigtails and tie a bandanna around your neck (this might come in handy later for light bondage). Then tell your lover (the experienced farmhand) to pretend he's teaching you the ins and outs of sex: where he likes to be touched or kissed, where he wants to kiss or touch you, and so on. Let him lead the way, and really try to pretend like you've never done this before.

Hot and spicy: This time, you play the naughty milkmaid, and he plays the farmer's shy and timid son. Dress the part of a milkmaid (think flowered dress and no undergarments) or the farm girl (overalls with nothing underneath). You lead him by the hand and show him all the details of the birds and the bees.

Up the Ante

- You play the role of the shy girl next door, and he plays the part of the horny teenager. Pretend you're shy and timid while he tries hard to seduce you. At some point in the game, drop the shy role and turn on your inner vixen!

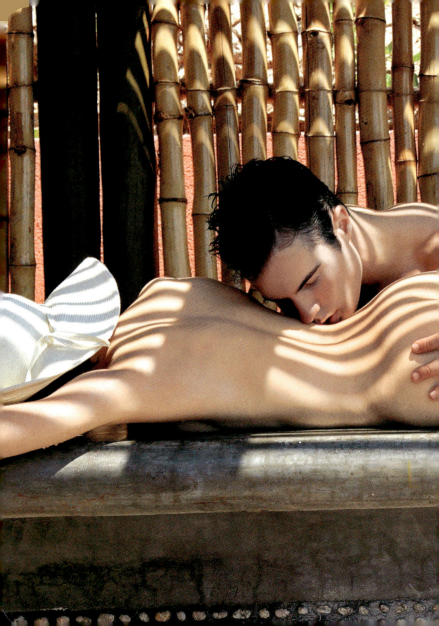

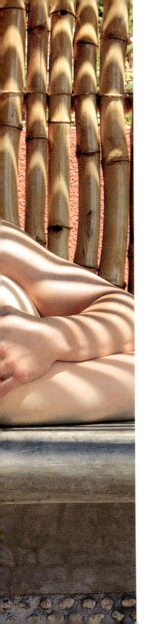

71

Pool Boy and Horny Housewife

Every woman loves imagining the fantasy of the hot, seductive pool boy who stops by while she's sunbathing (and the husband's far from home)!

The Sexy Setup

Tell your lover you have a fantasy game that's best played outdoors, near a pool or water.

Rules & Tools

Wear your sexiest bikini and your most seductive sandals. If you don't have a pool, set up a make-believe poolside setting: Drape a beach towel over your couch, serve some sexy summertime drinks, and get out the suntan lotion. Ask your lover to wear a summery shirt, shorts (or bathing suit), and flip-flops. Don't forget the sunglasses!

Playing the Game

Sweet and safe: You're the horny housewife who wants to get tan—all over. The problem is, you can't reach your back to apply the lotion, so you need his help. Lie on your stomach, untie your bikini top, and ask him to put suntan lotion on your backside. As he rubs you down, begin your seduction: Moan suggestively, arch your back, push your buttocks against him, or dangle your arm and rub his ankle suggestively.

Turn over suddenly, accidentally losing your top and exposing your breasts. Pretend to be surprised, but then tell him you like to sunbathe topless, and you'll need lotion on your front side as well!

Hot and spicy: Set yourself up as if you are sunbathing topless, but you're getting hornier and hornier as you watch him clean the pool (or move around the room). Start to touch yourself, then just lay back and start masturbating—but command him to keep cleaning the pool. See how long you can prevent him from joining in on some fun in the sun!

Up the Ante

- You're sunbathing nude, and he comes in to clean the pool. Act surprised, but then ask him if he minds if you stay undressed. Ask him to put lotion on your backside, but then send him away (to his make-believe cleaning task). Keep inviting him back, but play hard to get until he can't keep his hands off you!

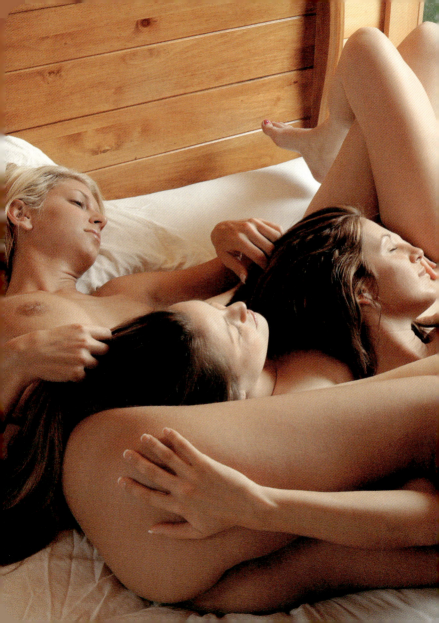

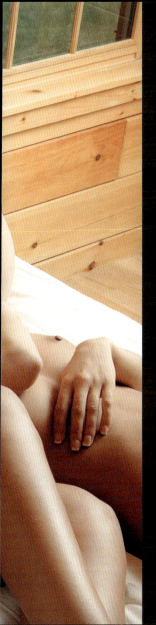

CHAPTER 7

Company's Coming
(Walk-ins Welcome)

If you've always wanted to add another player to your game, whether that involves another woman or another man, then this is the place for you. Try these games with all your favorite threesomes!

72

Sloppy
Seconds

This is a great beginning game for threesomes, or for women who aren't sure about being with another woman.

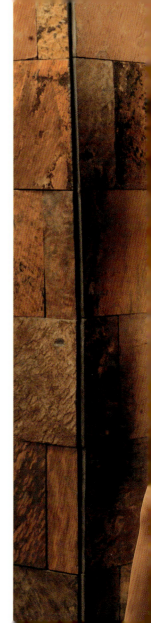

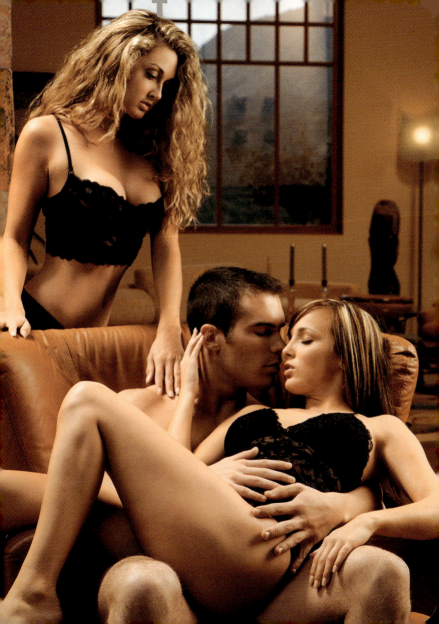

The Sexy Setup

Tell your female lover you have a game that involves one of her friends, but you're going to do all the work!

Rules & Tools

The rules can vary depending on how your lover feels about having her friend involved. Make sure you ask her what she's comfortable with, then plan the game accordingly.

Playing the Game

Sweet and safe: Ask both women to dress in their sexiest lingerie. Take your lover into your lap and kiss her passionately; the second female lover should just watch from afar. Cradle your lover in your lap and lavish her body with kisses and caresses, then slowly slip your fingers into her panties and bring her to orgasm. Don't let the second female masturbate—tell her she's got to wait her turn!

Hot and spicy: Have your female lover swap places with the second woman. She should be hot and wet at this point, so get right into her panties and find that clitoris. Have your first female lover watch—and masturbate, if needed.

Up the Ante

- Here's a great way to introduce your female lover to another woman's body: While the second woman is on your lap, have your female lover caress her breasts, touch her belly, or even kiss her feet, legs, and thighs.

- If you're playing this game with two men and one woman, let the first male lover have sex, then let the second male lover have sex with the female again.

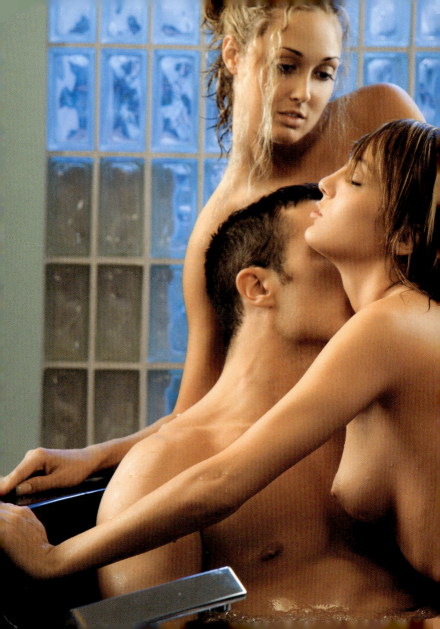

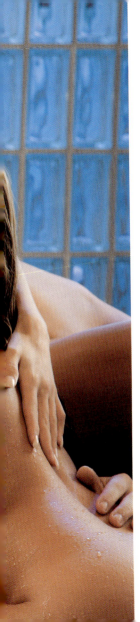

73

Ladies Locker-Room Fun

Here's another game for two girlfriends and their male lover. Call it *Girl, Interrupted*!

The Sexy Setup

Set up a time and place where you and your girlfriend can get naked and be alone, then arrange a time for your male lover to "accidentally" stumble in on the action.

Rules & Tools

This game works well in locations where females congregate and males aren't usually allowed—the ladies' locker room, the dressing room of a lingerie store, girls night out, etc. Or you can set the scene at home—it all depends on whether you're turned on by the possibility of getting caught!

Playing the Game

Sweet and safe: You and your girlfriend are in the ladies' locker room, showering up or enjoying a hot tub soak after a hard workout. Noticing that no one else is around, and that you're both completely naked, you start kissing and touching each other. Suddenly, your male lover walks in by accident! You keep at it, pretending you don't notice him, but watching your naked bodies together is a big turn-on, so he starts masturbating. Play out the game in whatever way brings the three of you the most pleasure.

Hot and spicy: You and your girlfriend are sharing one of the large, oversize dressing rooms at the local department store. (Look for a room where the walls go all the way to the ceiling for maximum privacy.) Bring a variety of sexy lingerie into the dressing room, and take turns trying things on and modeling things for each other. Suddenly, someone knocks at the door, and in comes your male lover! Continue the lingerie show for him, but add in some touching and kissing between the two of you to get him heated up. Once he's hard, sit behind him and kiss and nuzzle his neck while your girlfriend continues modeling. Rub his chest, and as he gets hard, reach around from behind and fondle his penis. Let your girlfriend continue the modeling show while you give him a hand job he'll never forget!

Up the Ante

- Sit behind him, and have him lean back against your breasts. His hands can fondle your buttocks or thighs while your hands stroke his chest and belly. Have your girlfriend come in close and stimulate him orally. Once he's hard, have her ride him like a cowgirl while the two of you fondle her breasts!

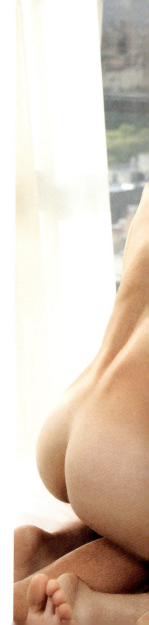

74

Oreo Cookie
(and You're the Filling!)

This game is designed for two men and one woman. The idea: sandwich her from either side like an Oreo cookie, and she's the yummy filling!

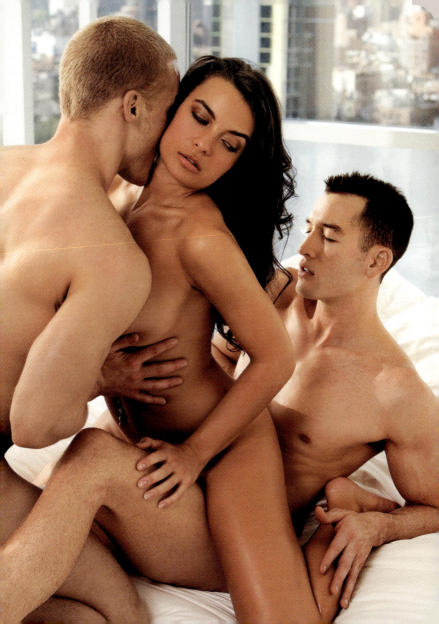

The Sexy Setup

Tell your lover that you want to maximize her pleasure—
you and another male friend are going to worship her body
and give her all the pleasure she can take.

Rules & Tools

This is a game designed for pleasuring the female; it's
perfect for women who aren't that comfortable with sexual
contact between two men. Decide which of you wants to
"service" her front side, and which of you wants to play
"backdoor man."

Playing the Game

Sweet and safe: This is a simple game of two on one.
She sits back and does nothing but orgasm, while you two
sandwich her from either side. Start by undressing her
with one of you facing her front (and kissing her passionately), while the other works from the rear. As you undress
her, focus on her front side—touch her breasts, nuzzle her
neck, and kiss her belly. Your backside partner should do
the same: Kiss the small of her back, fondle her backside,
and caress her thighs.

Ultimately, the front side lover should manually or orally stimulate her clitoris in order to bring her to orgasm while the backside partner spoons her from behind, fondles her from behind, and squeezes her nipples. Having two sets of hands all over her body is sure to drive her crazy!

Hot and spicy: Turn up the action. While you kiss and fondle her from the front side, have your backside partner enter her from behind. Once he's thrusting in and out, move down and stimulate her clitoris orally. She won't know whether she's coming or going!

Up the Ante

- Stimulate her orally, but have your backside partner stimulate her anus with a set of anal beads.

- For the ultimate four-prong orgasm, kiss her deeply while stimulating her clitoris manually. Have your backside partner enter her from behind and insert a finger into her anus. Every orifice accounted for!

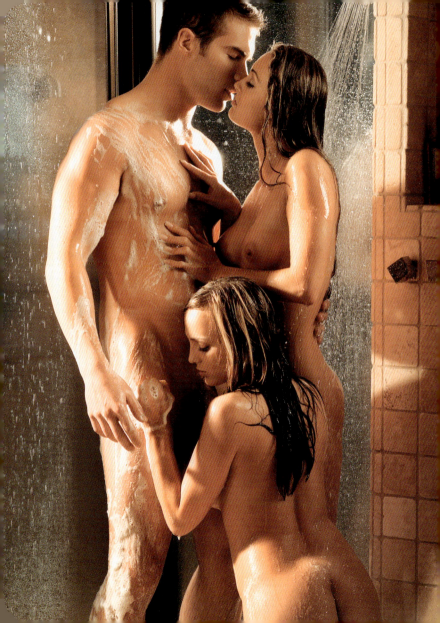

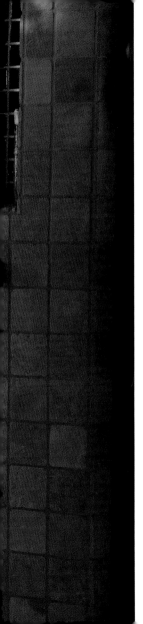

75

Merry Go Round

Here's a game where everybody's giving—
and receiving—pleasure. It works best
for two women and a male lover, but you
can switch to two men and a woman
if everyone's comfortable.

The Sexy Setup

Tell your female lover you want to hook up with her and one of her sexiest friends (she can pick who she wants to join you). Then ask if she prefers to be a giver or a taker—either role is fine with you.

Rule & Tools

There are two roles in this game: the lover who gives pleasure, and the lover who receives it. The goal is to have everyone playing both roles at once.

Playing the Game

Sweet and safe: Take turns kissing, touching, and undressing among the three of you until everyone is naked. Then suggest you all take a shower together, where the steam and heat can help everyone relax. Stand up, kiss your female lover, and finger her clitoris while her girlfriend sucks on you and masturbates at the same time. Alternatively, have your lover stand up while you kiss her genitals and clitoris; she can kiss and finger her girlfriend while you masturbate.

Hot and spicy: Move to the bed for this action. Lie down, and ask your female lover to sit on your face, facing your feet. Have her girlfriend climb on you cowgirl style. You stimulate your lover orally while the two girls kiss and fondle each other's breasts. The second woman rides you to orgasm!

Up the Ante

- Have one of the two female lovers lie down. Kneel over her in a classic 69 so she can suck you off. You stimulate the second woman orally while she fingers her girlfriend's clitoris!

- Let everyone find a penis or clitoris to touch, suck, lick, and stimulate—then try to orgasm simultaneously!

76

Three of a Kind

Here's a game that's perfectly suited for three women. Call it anything you want, but remember that three of a kind beats any pair!

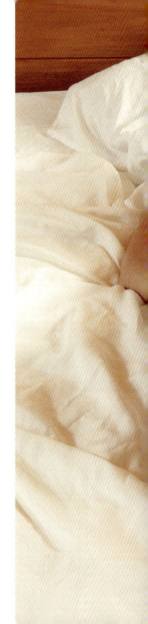

The Sexy Setup

Tell your female lover you want to treat her to something special—another flavor of pussy. Then whisper just how hot you get thinking about six sets of nipples and three clits all playing together!

Rules & Tools

The name of this game is pleasure, and it's all about reveling in the female body. You'll need a blindfold and something for restraining one of your lovers.

Playing the Game

Sweet and safe: Pick one woman to be the receiver, and the other two play givers. Blindfold and tie the receiver to the bed, then take turns kissing her all over. One of you can caress her breasts and nipples while the other licks her way downward to the inner thighs, labia, and clitoris. When you bring her to orgasm, have one of you focus on her nipples while the other concentrates on her clitoris.

Hot and spicy: Lie in a circle, using each other's legs as pillows, and stimulate each other orally. Run your hands up and down your lover's body, taking time to squeeze her nipples, caress her breasts, and fondle her buttocks. This is great fun because everyone's giving **and** getting pleasure!

Up the Ante

- Form a circle of three (described in hot and spicy) but introduce some toys into the circle: Use an anal vibrator on one of you, a dildo on the second, and nipple clamps on the third. Set a timer and switch toys (and positions!).

- Have one woman restrain the second, then both work on the third together. Swap roles after you've rocked her world.

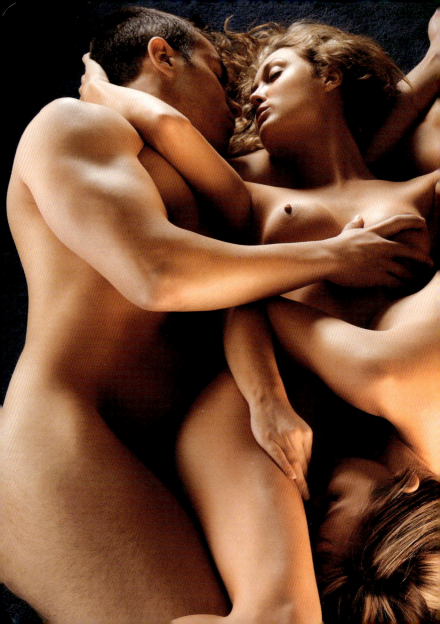

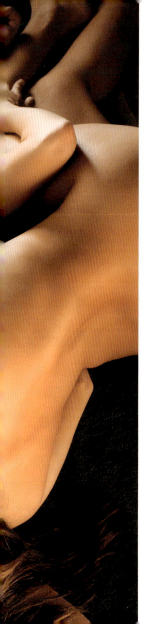

77

Daisy Chain

This game is based on the most famous three-way position out there, and it's versatile to boot—it accommodates two women and one male lover or two men and one woman.

The Sexy Setup

Tell your male lover you have a little surprise for him: a game of daisy chain. If he doesn't know what this means, all the better—he's in for a special treat!

Rules & Tools

Take turns with who's in the middle and everyone will love this game.

Playing the Game

Sweet and safe (for two women and one man):

Take turns kissing, touching, and undressing the three of you until everyone is naked—and hot! Lie down, and have your male lover spoon you from behind. Turn to kiss him, exposing your breasts and nipples for stimulation, or present your backside in full and let him enter you from behind as you turn your face toward your female lover's genitals and enter into a female variation of 69.

Hot and spicy (for two men and one woman): Take turns kissing, touching, and undressing the three of you until everyone is naked, hot, and wet. Lie on your side and ask your male lover to spoon you from behind. Turn and kiss him deeply and let him caress your breasts, nipples, and belly. Ask your second male lover to stimulate you orally. Be prepared for a two-pronged orgasm!

Up the Ante

- Lie on your side, and have your first male lover penetrate you anally while your second male lover enters your vagina. Alternatively, have the second lover use a dildo in your vagina and stimulate your clitoris manually. Chances are this three-pronged pleasure will bring you to orgasm in record time!

78
Queen of the Stairs

Want to play queen for a day?
Try this game on the stairs for better
access to all your hidden treasures.

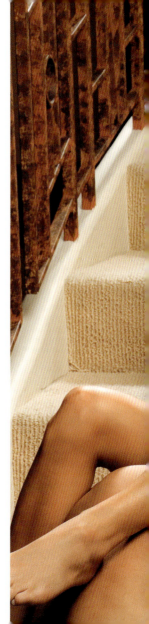

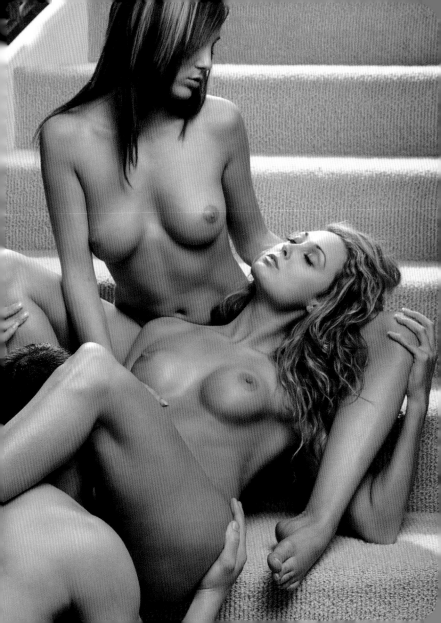

The Sexy Setup

Tell your female lover you want to worship her body, and you're bringing along a sex slave (male or female) for assistance.

Rules & Tools

This game is best played on the stairs, where the height variations give you better access to your female lover's assets. What's more, you'll get the best seat in the house for watching her writhe with pleasure!

Playing the Game

Sweet and safe: Take turns kissing, touching, and undressing your female lover between the two of you until she's hot and wet. Sit down on the stairs, and cradle her head in your lap. Caress her breasts, squeeze her nipples, and hold her down while he stimulates her orally. Be prepared to masturbate if you can't control yourself!

Hot and spicy: With your female lover's head in your lap, have her suck on your nipples and caress your breasts. Reach down and stimulate her clitoris manually, but have your male lover penetrate her from a lower step.

Up the Ante

- Make yourself the queen of the stairs. Sit back, and ask your female lover to turn around and stimulate your clitoris orally. Ask your male lover to flip on his back and stimulate her orally from underneath or kneel behind her, lean over and grab her breasts, and do her doggie style.

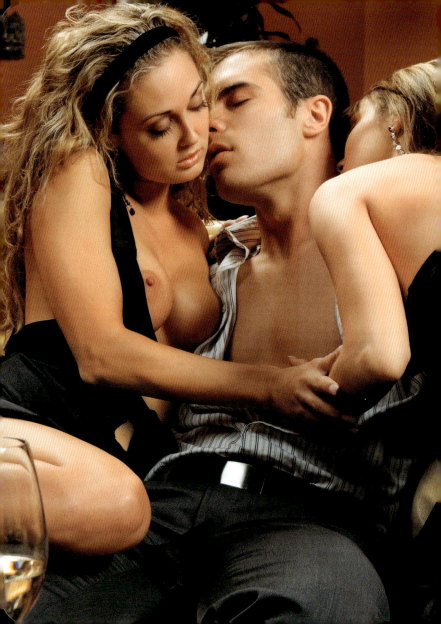

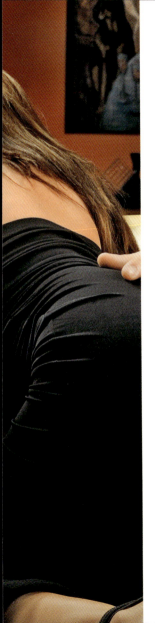

79

Twin Sisters

This is a fun and sassy guessing game for a pair of women and their male lover. Satisfaction guaranteed!

The Sexy Setup

Tell your male lover that you and your girlfriend are pretending to be twin sisters. He's been dating one of you, but the second sister has secretly gone on several dates with him (or had sex!) and so far he hasn't noticed. He has to try and guess which of you is which!

Rules & Tools

You'll need a blindfold for your male lover (sweet and safe) as well as restraints (hot and spicy).

Playing the Game

Sweet and safe: Blindfold your lover, and tell him he's being worked on by twin sisters. Whenever you ask, he must try to guess whose hands, mouth, or body parts he's in contact with. Start by undressing him very slowly; one can kiss him passionately while the other unbuttons his shirt or removes his pants, then swap places. Once he's completely naked, alternate between one of you kissing him while the other stimulates him orally. Make your swapping as seamless as possible, and mirror each other as you let him touch your breasts or buttocks.

Hot and spicy: Take it up a notch by securing his hands and feet to the bed or couch where you're playing. Take turns letting him suck your nipples or kiss your breasts while your girlfriend goes down on him, then swap. As things heat up, sit on his face and let him nuzzle your genitals while she rides him in the cowgirl position, then swap again. The goal—to keep him guessing while stimulating every sense possible!

Up the Ante

- When he's ready to come, join forces at his penis. One of you can lick or fondle the shaft while the other sucks on the head. Remember, twin sisters do everything together—even making their lover come!

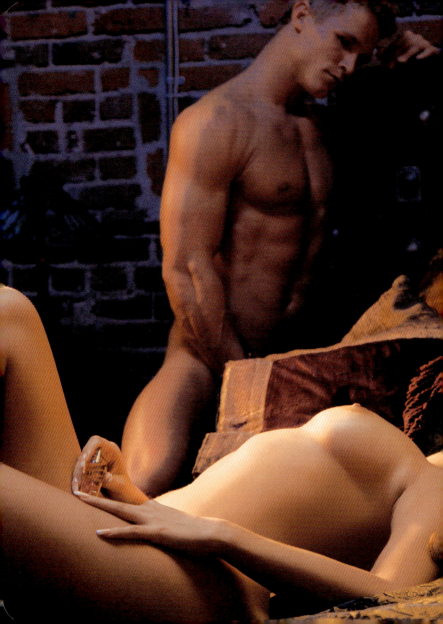

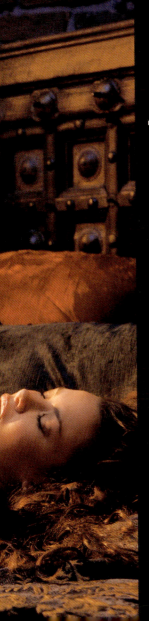

CHAPTER 8

Toys and Props

Interested in toys and props? These devices can take your sex play to a new and different level of satisfaction! Although these games are designed specifically for using toys, remember that any sex toy can find a place in any game, so let your imagination soar—and enjoy the sensations!

80

Remote Control

If you like to tease your partner all night long before delivering the goods, this game of remote control pleasure is a perfect fit!

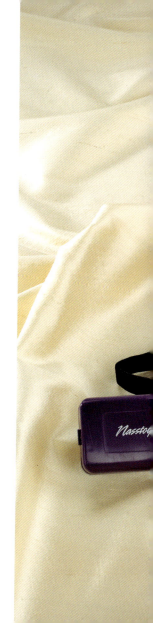

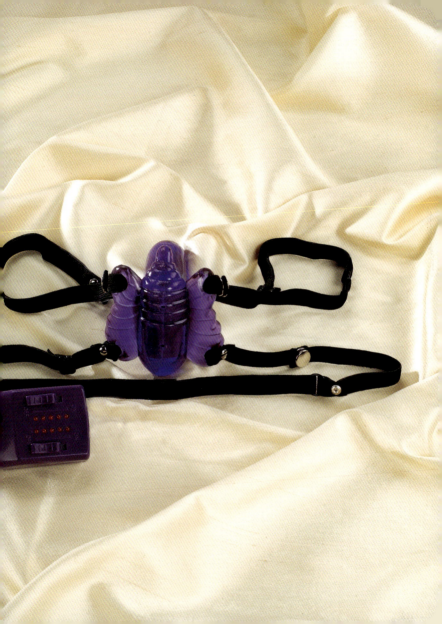

The Sexy Setup

Plan a night out on the town, perhaps a romantic dinner followed by dancing at a club or playing pool at the local pub. Tell your lover you're footing the bill, but in return she has to wear a special something under her skirt.

Rules & Tools

Purchase a fluttering butterfly-style clitoral stimulator with a wireless remote control.

Playing the Game

Sweet and safe: Present the butterfly to your lover in a specially wrapped box, and ask her to wear it under her skirt. When she asks what it does, tell her she'll find out as the night progresses. Take your lover to dinner, buy her a drink, and use the remote control to give her a tiny buzz. She should be pleasantly surprised! Continue buzzing her from time to time throughout your dinner while you play footsie or gaze deeply into her eyes. If this is her first time wearing one of these devices, consider bringing her to orgasm in a semiprivate place, such as a dark alley or your car, then give her time to recover.

Hot and spicy: Take it up a notch by buzzing her throughout the night, but bring her closer to the brink of orgasm and then stop. Once you're out on the dance floor at the club, bring her over the top in time to the pulsating music, or hold her close during a slow dance and let her climax. Chances are no one will hear her moans of pleasure or notice her quivering legs with all the music and dancing!

Up the Ante

- Once she's hot and wet, whisk her into a darkened hallway or unused bedroom and give her a double-pronged orgasm: Enter her from behind and hit the on button. Aim for perfectly timed orgasms together!

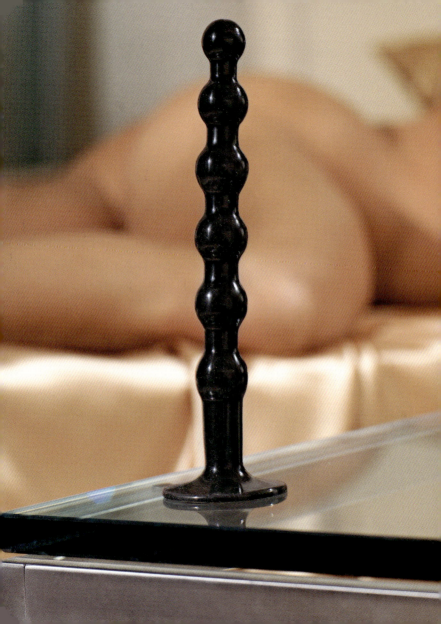

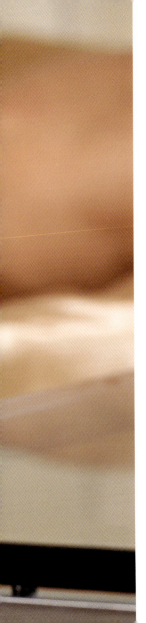

81

Pleasure Party

If you've ever attended one of those female-only pleasure parties to purchase sex toys, you'll recognize the roots of this naughty game!

The Sexy Setup

Invite your lover to a "pleasure party" designed for two.
Tell him you have a special lineup of tools and tricks to
bring him hours of delight.

Rules & Tools

Set a sexy and sensuous setting: Build a nest of blankets
and furs on the floor, light some candles, and put on your
sexiest lingerie. Line up all your sex toys, but keep them
hidden under a silky scarf.

Playing the Game

Sweet and safe: Welcome your lover with a long and lin-
gering kiss, then undress him partially and ask him to get
comfortable. Tell him you're the mistress of pleasure and
you're going to demonstrate all the different tools. One by
one, bring out your sex toys and use them on various parts
of his body, building tension and heightening the excitement
as you go. Use a vibrator to massage his neck and shoulders, then buzz his nipples gently with a vibrating finger
device. Move down his body and tickle his perineum or
around his testicles with your device as you stroke his penis.

Use each device to turn him on for a bit, but don't bring him to orgasm—stop and introduce the next toy until he's ready to burst! Then help him climax in whatever way feels best!

Hot and spicy: Help your lover undress completely, and invite him into the pleasure nest. Show him all your toys, but then blindfold him and tie his hands above his head. Tell him he must guess the toy in question as you use it on his body. If he guesses correctly you'll reward him with a kiss (or a sip of champagne, bite of chocolate, etc.), but if he guesses incorrectly he might get a spank or a gentle slap. Test your toys one by one and think creatively: Use your vibrating devices on different areas of his body, slip on a cock ring and ride him for a few minutes, then jump off and insert his penis into a sleeve. Keep him guessing until he can't hold back!

Up the Ante

- Try multiple toys at once: Insert a string of anal beads, then press your bullet vibrator against the base of his penis while you suck him off. Pull out the beads just as he climaxes!

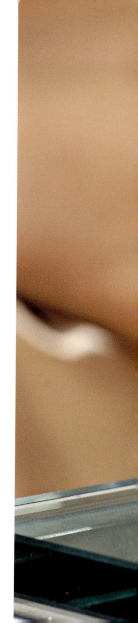

82

Backdoor Woman

You've heard the phrase "backdoor man"? This time the roles are reversed: You get to control the action at your male lover's back door!

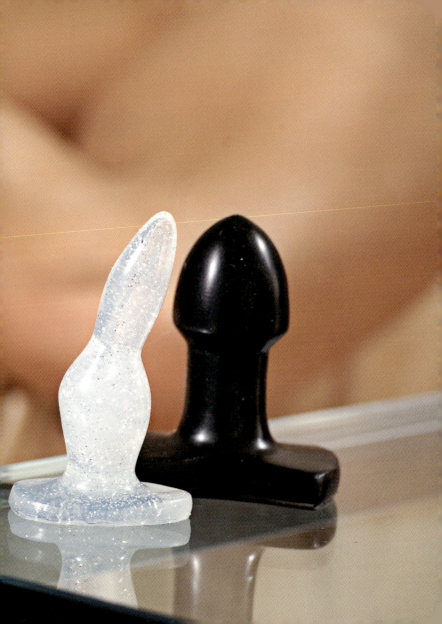

The Sexy Setup

Write your male lover a sexy note and tell him you want to explore his back door. Promise you'll be gentle as you investigate his backside assets, but you're sure there are some new pleasures zones worth exploring!

Rules & Tools

You'll want to line up a number of anal toys for this game, and plenty of lubrication. Have these (or other toys) on hand: butt plug, strap-on dildo, anal vibrator, anal beads, or any pocket-size or finger vibrator. Set up a low-lit, sexy scene for this game, and line a couch with fur, create a nest of soft blankets on the floor, or make up your bed with silk sheets.

Playing the Game

Sweet and safe: If this is your lover's first time with anal play, take it slow. Dress in your sexiest lingerie and help him loosen up by serving him a drink. Then take out your toys and let him look at them close up. Explain why you think each one might turn him on, but be open if he's not interested.

Kiss and caress him in your usual way, then slowly move to fondling and sucking his penis and nibbling his testicles. Try running a finger vibrator along his inner thighs, up to his testicles, and along his perineum. Be sure to ask if he likes the feeling, and if he does, continue with your backdoor play, perhaps inserting the butt plug or anal beads while you suck him off.

Hot and spicy: You know your man's open to any anal suggestion, so take it up a notch and explore your own fantasies. Lube up the strap-on dildo and give it to him up the ass like the strong and sexy backdoor woman you are, or just insert a vibrating butt plug and ride him like a cowgirl!

Up the Ante

- Play a game of "Backdoor Woman Meets Backdoor Man." Both of you should choose your favorite butt plug, then have intercourse doggie style!

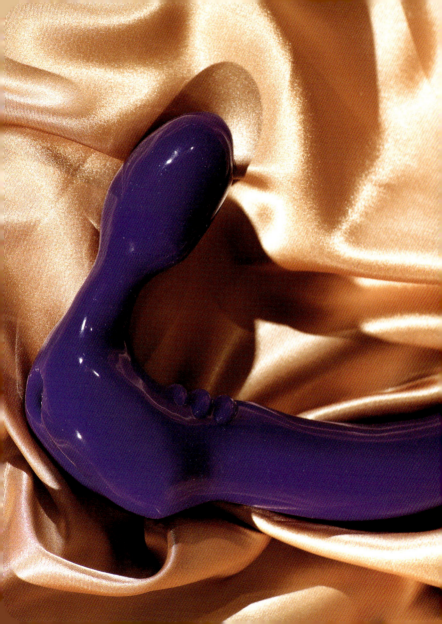

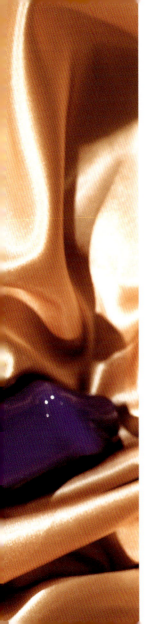

83

Good Vibrations

This is a perfect game for treating your female lover to a night of pleasure, all of it involving good vibrations!

The Sexy Setup

Text your lover and tell her you have a special night planned, and the theme is good vibrations. Chances are just that suggestion will get her hot under the hood!

Rules & Tools

Set a sexy scene for your night of pleasure: Build a fire, turn the lights down low, and put on some sensuous music. Have a blindfold ready and line up all your toys that vibrate, whether that's the cone, a miniature clit vibrator, or something in between. Remember, this game is about using a variety of vibrators to tantalize every inch of your lover's body!

Playing the Game

Sweet and safe: Slowly undress your lover; kiss her deeply, and run your hands all over her body, telling her just how hot and sexy she is. Blindfold her and lead her to the vibrating pleasure zone. Start out slowly, perhaps using a vibrating wand on her neck and shoulders. Try a different vibrating device on various body parts: Massage her muscles with long smooth strokes, tickle her nipples with a vibrating finger device, and finally move to her genitals.

Here you can use a vibrator to tease open her labia, switch gears to reach her G-spot, and then come back to her clitoris for the final climax!

Hot and spicy: Take it up a notch: Use a pair of vibrating nipple clips to keep her on her toes while you insert a vibrating butt plug or have her grind on a cone-like device. Once she's hot and wet, turn on that U-shaped vibrator and stimulate her G-spot and her clitoris at the same time. Let her ride the vibrations to heaven and back!

Up the Ante

- Pick two or three of your favorite vibrating devices, and start at her toes. Moving very, very slowly, use each device on every inch of her, taking care to test every speed, pulsation, and pattern. Keep her guessing where you're going next and what it will feel like, and build the tension by avoiding the genitals until her clitoris is fully engorged!

84

Finger Fun

Here's a game for men or women—
just let your fingers do the talking!

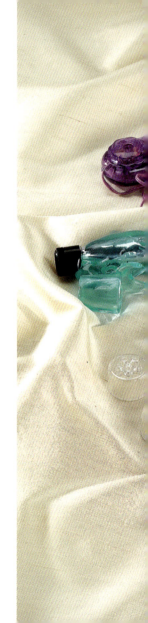

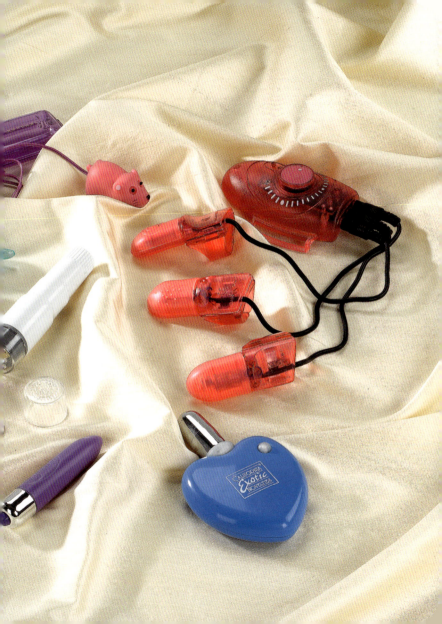

The Sexy Setup

Call your lover and tell her you have some fingers that are itching to do some exploring, and some toys that will add to the fun!

Rules & Tools

You'll need an assortment of finger toys or some miniature vibrators for this game.

Playing the Game

Sweet and safe: Kiss your lover passionately, nuzzle her neck, and slowly undress her with both hands. Have her lie down or get comfortable in a sofa chair, and arm yourself with your finger toys or miniature vibrators. Starting at her toes, tickle her every fantasy. Lick her toes while you finger her labia, then move up to nibble her thighs while you stimulate her clitoris. Add some tongue action and move the finger toy to her nipples—she'll be begging for more!

Hot and spicy: Get your lover hot and wet, then ask her to kneel on all fours so you can enter her from behind. Reach around her front side with your finger vibrator in place and stimulate her clitoris. Try to time your climaxes together!

Up the Ante

- Ask your lover to suck you off and use the finger vibrator on your perineum or testicles. Satisfaction guaranteed!

- Have your lover ride you cowgirl style, but stimulate her nipples with the finger vibrators.

- Ask your lover to stimulate *your* nipples or other erogenous zones with the finger vibrators.

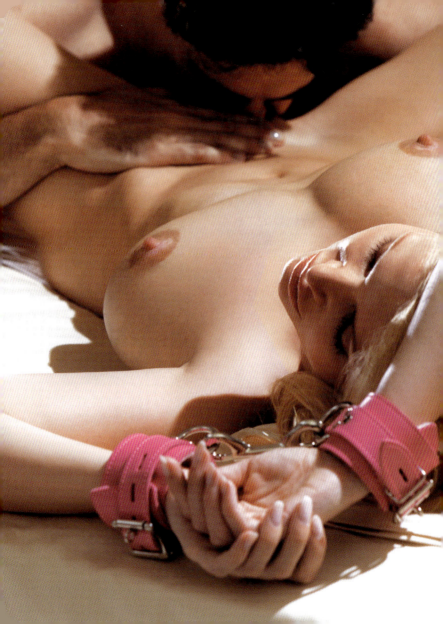

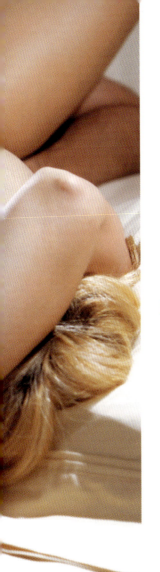

85

Tie and Tease

Want to give your female lover the added time and attention she deserves? Try this game of tie and tease and prooooooolong her pleasure!

The Sexy Setup

Send your lover a note or leave a sexy voice mail and tell her you know she's been working hard and feeling underappreciated. You have a night of pleasure designed to help her unwind—and you'll do all the work!

Rules & Tools

Get a set of handcuffs or rope, a blindfold, and leg restraints, if desired. Line up your favorite lubrications, sex toys, feathers, and other good devices for teasing. Set a sexy scene by building a fire in the fireplace and creating a luxurious and sensual spot for her to lie. Ask her to wear a sexy outfit of her choosing, or buy her a new outfit—every woman loves presents!

Playing the Game

Sweet and safe: When she comes into the room, greet her with a deep, passionate kiss, and tell her how sexy she is. Serve her a drink, then lead her over to the pleasure zone. Gently restrain her hands, and tell her that her job is to lie back and enjoy the ride.

Once she's restrained, it's your turn to tease her as long as you like. Focus on her breasts and work slowly: Fondle and caress her breasts, squeeze and suck on her nipples. Next, move to her buttocks, then her thighs, and finally her genitals. If you draw out the teasing sufficiently, she may climax as soon as you touch her clitoris!

Hot and spicy: Restrain her legs, and add a blindfold. Use your favorite toys as you tease her mercilessly: Use nipple clamps while you kiss her inner thighs, insert a vibrating butt plug as you explore her labia with your fingers, or use your tongue around and around her clitoris while you insert a dildo in her vagina. Stimulate each area, but then move away before she even comes close to climaxing—the idea is to prolong the pleasure as long as possible and tease her into a mind-blowing orgasm!

Up the Ante

- Set up a video camera and film the teasing show. Play it back for her later, after she's climaxed, and get her hot and wet. Take her in any position you desire!

- Invite a second lover to help out in the game: The dual sensations, especially if she's blindfolded, will have her screaming for release!

Resources

www.adameve.com

www.afroerotik.com

www.allaboutthepenis.com

www.babeland.com

www.blowfish.com

www.bluedoor.com

www.clitical.com

www.comeasyouare.com

www.devinetoys.com

www.embodytantra.com

www.evesgarden.com

www.freddyandeddy.com

www.goodvibes.com

www.hiddenself.com

www.libida.com

www.mypleasure.com

www.purplepassion.com

www.sexinfo101.com

www.sexuality.org

www.sheerglydedams.com

www.sliptongue.com

www.sliquid.com

www.smittenkittenonline.com

www.stockroom.com

www.tinynibbles.com

www.wildinsecret.com

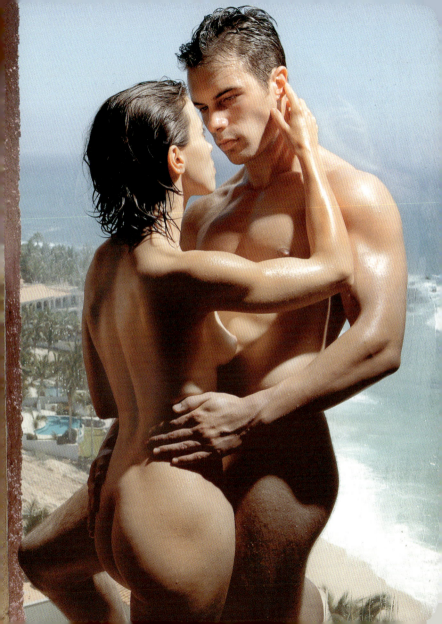

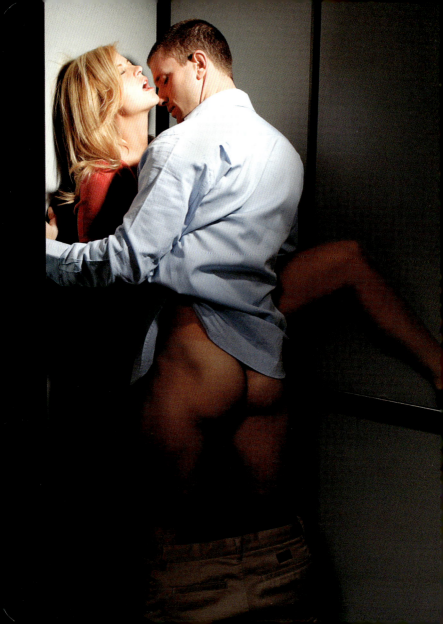

Your Checklist

How many have you
accomplished? Check
them off as you go!

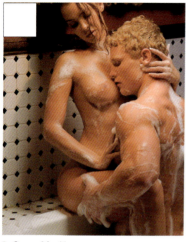

1 Soap Me Up

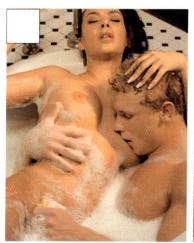

2 Preheat the Oven

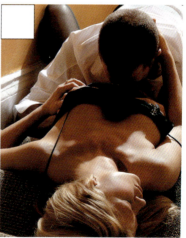

3 Tubby Time

4 Stair Climber

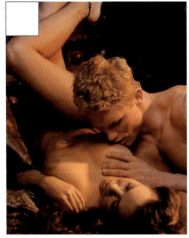

5 Fashion Show

6 Strip Poker

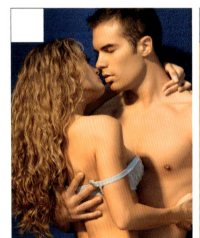

7 Strip Scrabble

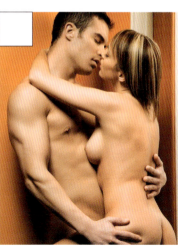

8 Strip Monopoly

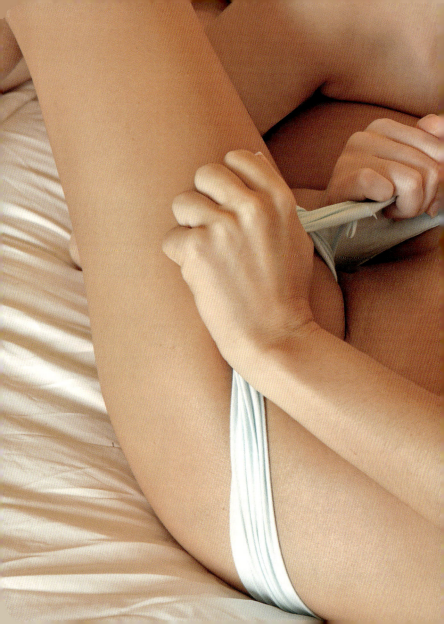

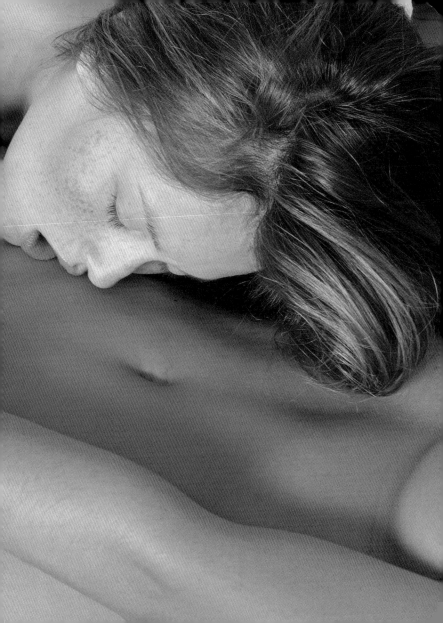

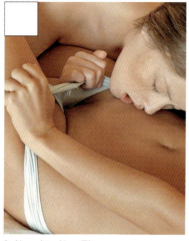

9 Naughty Nap Time

10 Movie Night

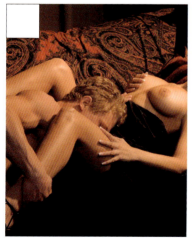

11 Blue Velvet

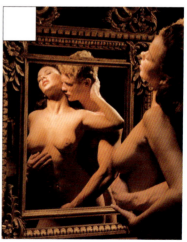

12 Anatomy Lessons

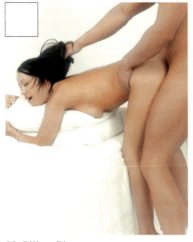

13 Pillow Pleasures

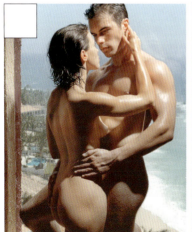

15 Talk It Up

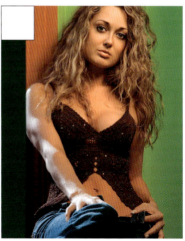

14 Show and Tell

16 Striptease

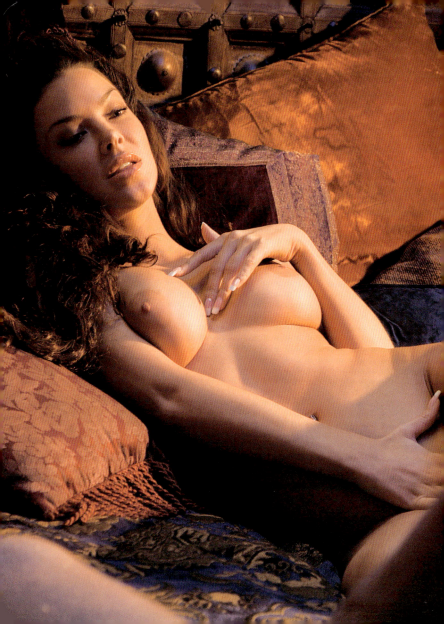

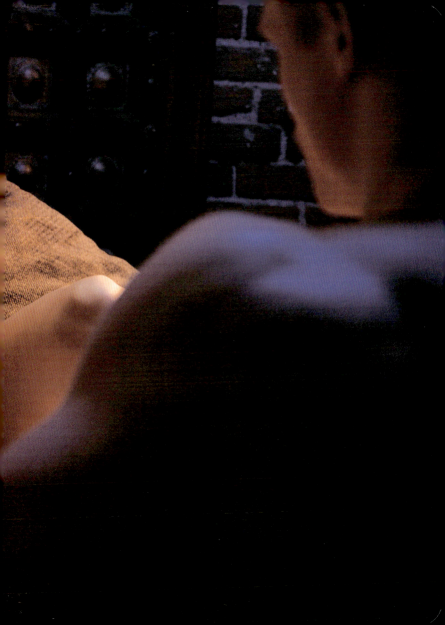

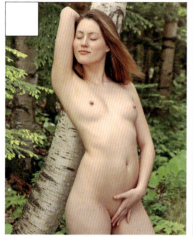

17 "Horny on Line One"

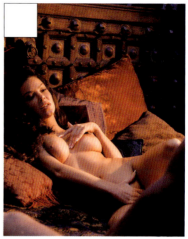

18 Pretty in Pearls

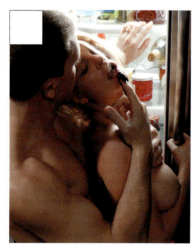

19 Make Me Your Own Sundae

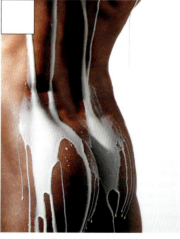

20 Milky Spa Bath

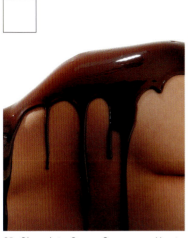

21 Chocolate Syrup Scavenger Hunt

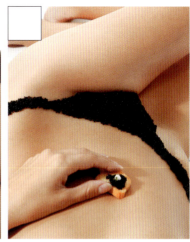

22 Picnic by Candlelight

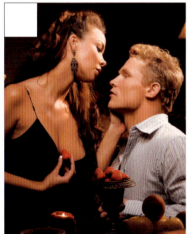

23 What's in the Fridge?

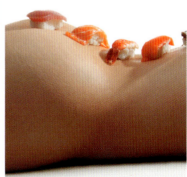

24 Naked Sushi

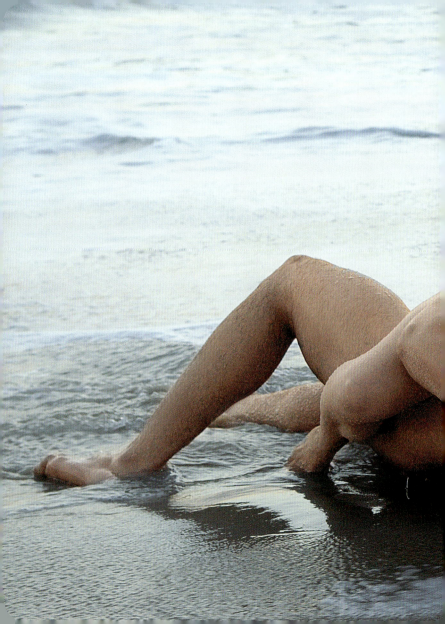

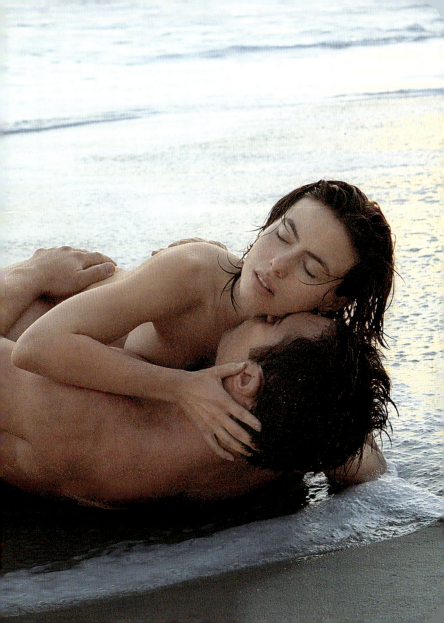

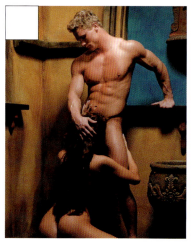

25 Peppermint Tingler

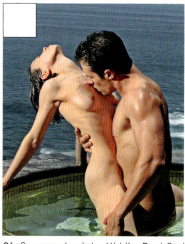

26 Summer Lovin'—Kiddie–Pool Style

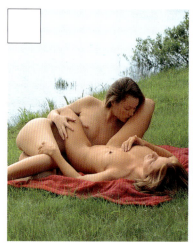

27 Lakeshore Loving

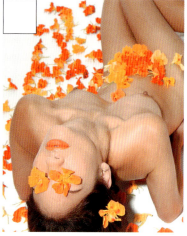

28 Bed of Flowers

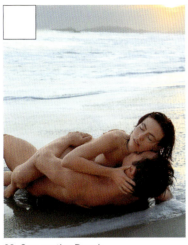

29 Sex on the Beach

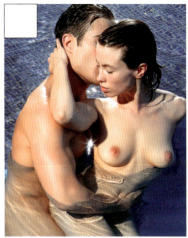

30 Poolside Pussy

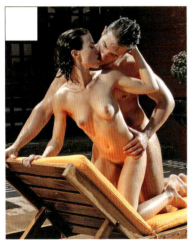

31 Lounge Chair Lovin'

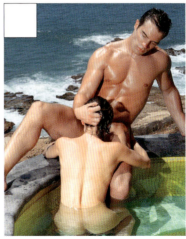

32 Hot Times in the Hot Tub

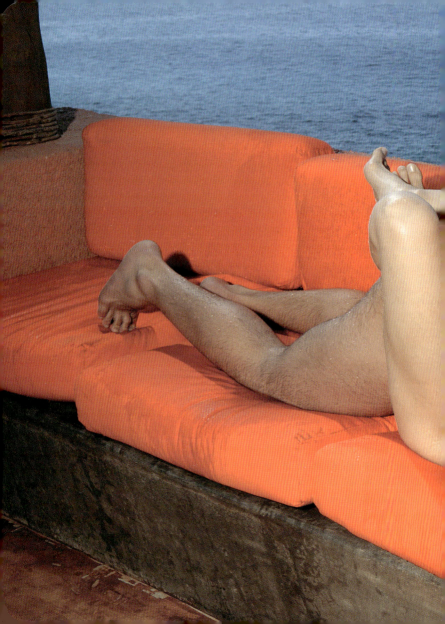

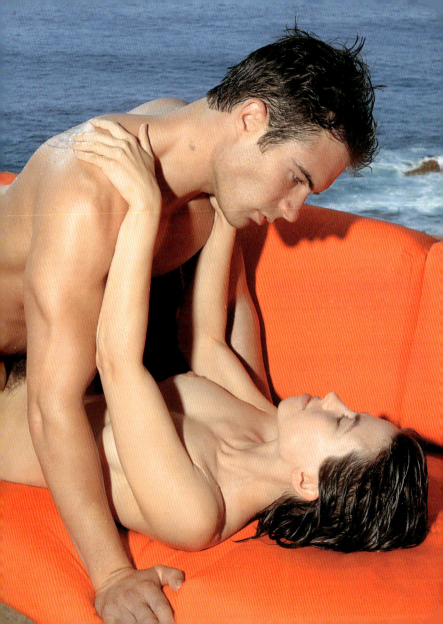

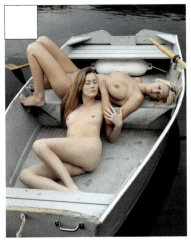

33 Ride the Waves (in a Boat!)

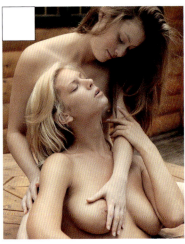

34 Playin' on the Playground

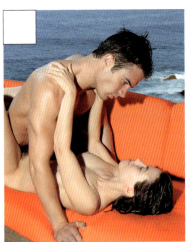

35 Missionary Man

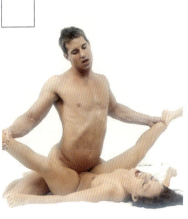

36 Get on Your Knees

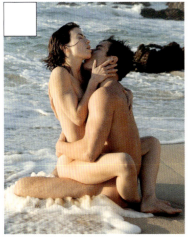

37 In the Lap of Luxury

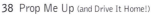

38 Prop Me Up (and Drive It Home!)

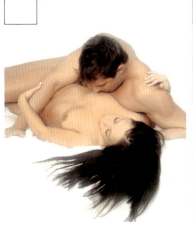

39 Spoonful of Lovin'

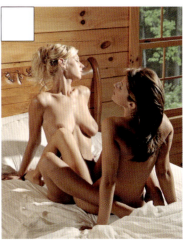

40 Scissors of Love

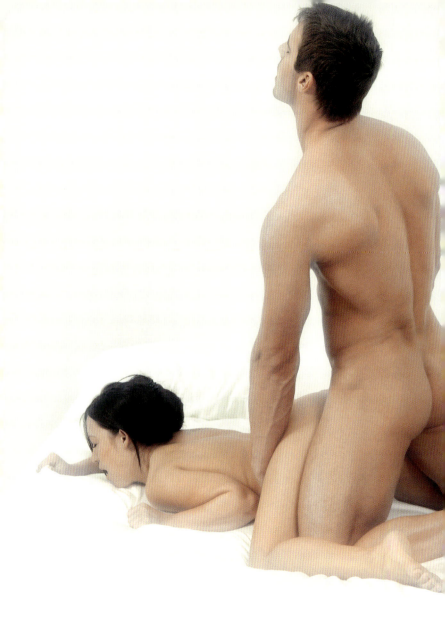

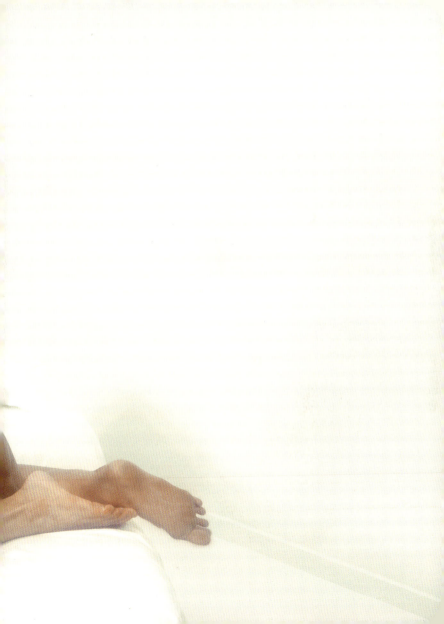

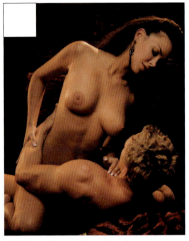

41 Cowgirl and Bucking Bronco

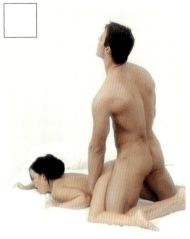

42 Doggie Style

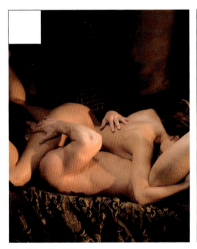

43 Classic 69

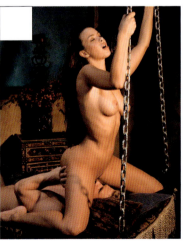

44 Sit on My Face

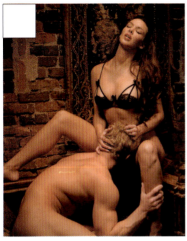

45 Seat of Honor

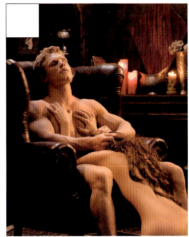

46 At Your Service

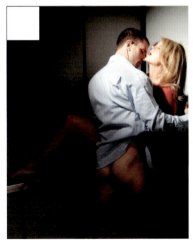

47 Going Down, Anyone?

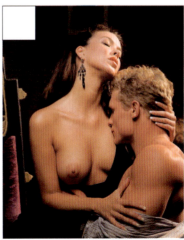

48 Ridin' the Rails

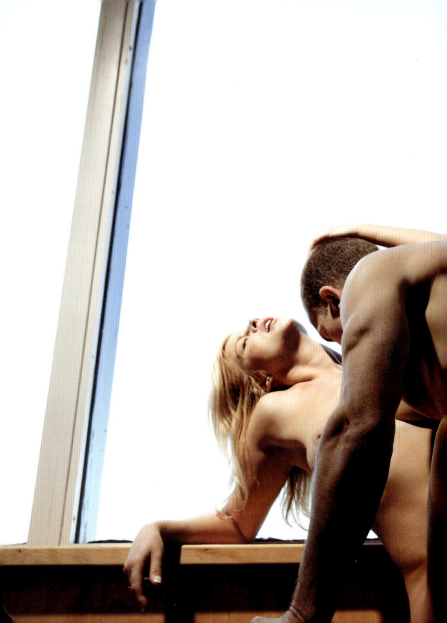

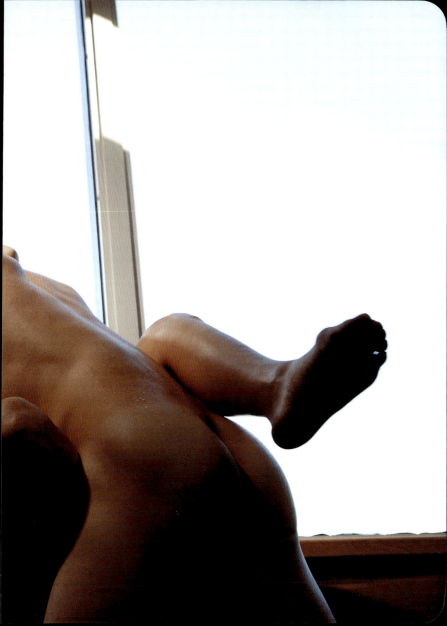

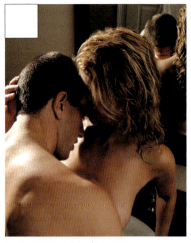

49 Restroom Rendezvous

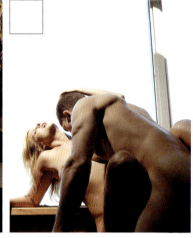

50 Mile High Club

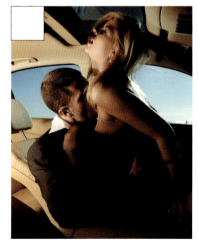

51 Auto-Erotica

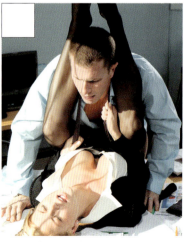

52 Hold My Calls (and My Balls!)

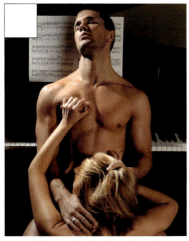

53 Frisky Fun in the Furniture Store

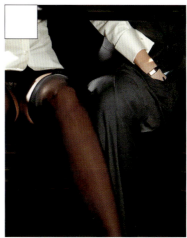

54 Movie Theater Hand Games

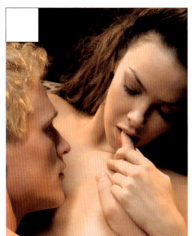

55 Let's Hear That Engine Purr

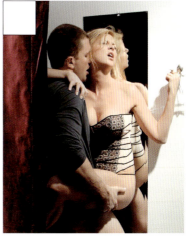

56 The Un-Dressing Room

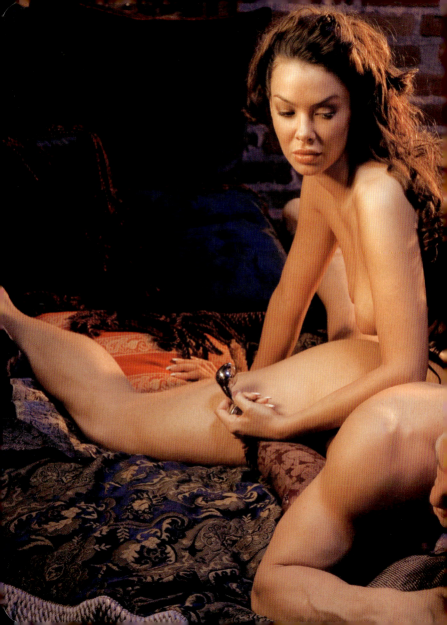

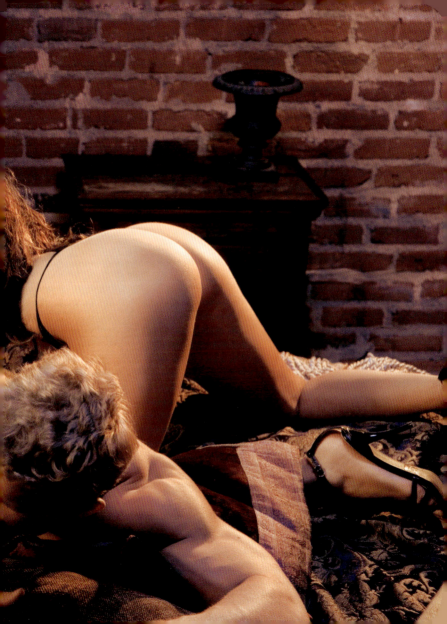

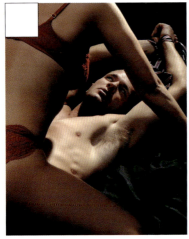

57 Sex in Space

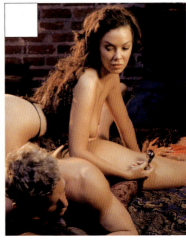

58 Door-to-Door Vibrator Salesman

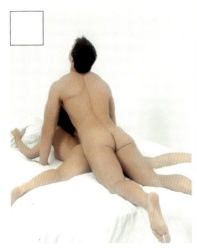

59 Under House Arrest

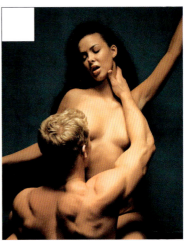

60 Flirty Flight Attendant

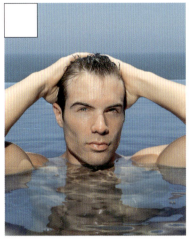

61 Handyman Cum Calling

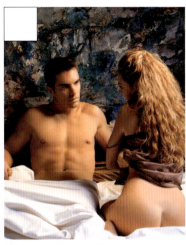

62 Horny Housemaid

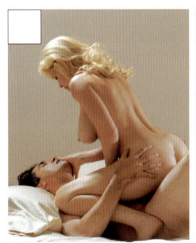

63 Visiting Nurse

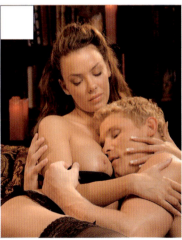

64 Pirate and Captive Maiden

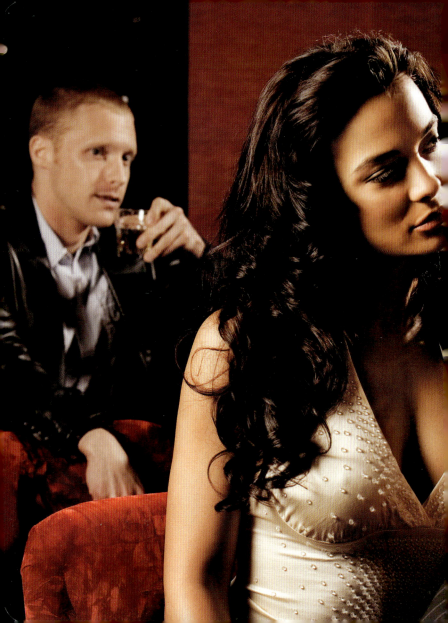

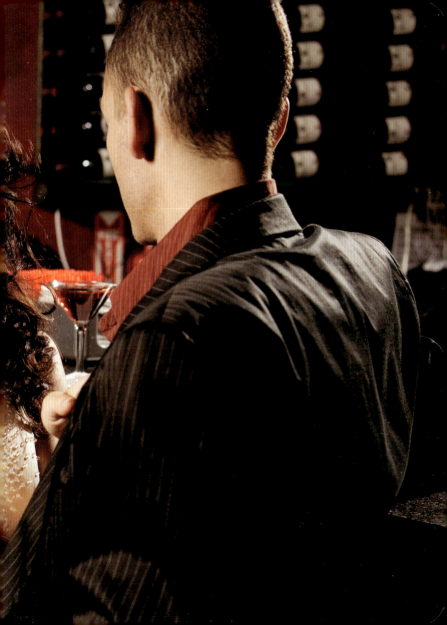

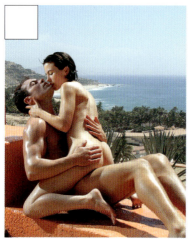

65 Mistress (or Master) and Sex Slave

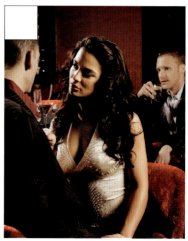

66 Pickup at the Bar

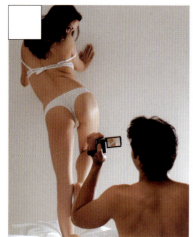

67 Porn Star and Director

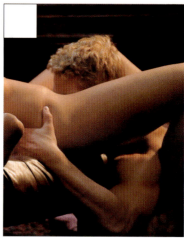

68 Surprise Sex

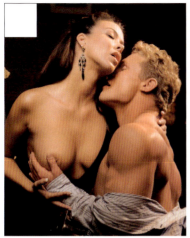
69 Hooker and Client

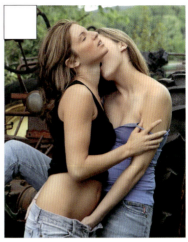
70 Farm Girl in the Hay

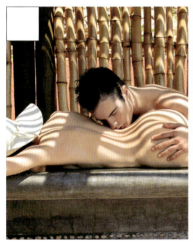
71 Pool Boy and Horny Housewife

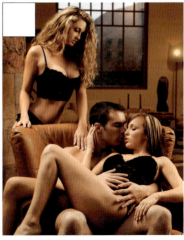
72 Sloppy Seconds

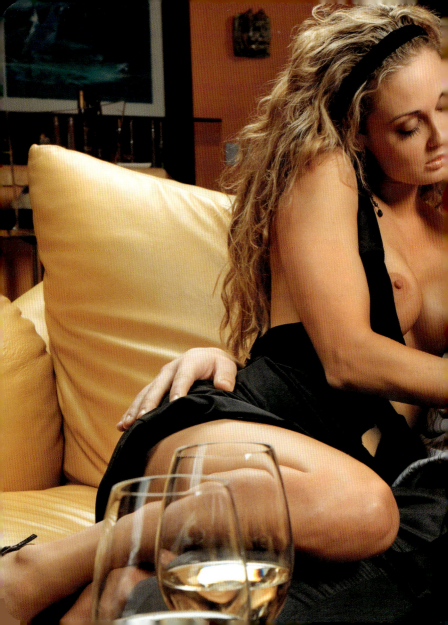

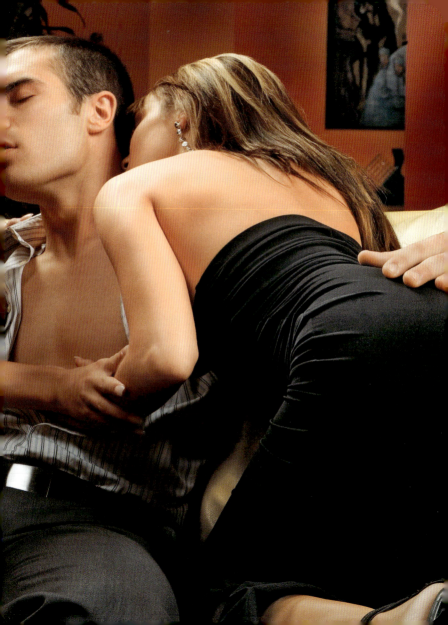

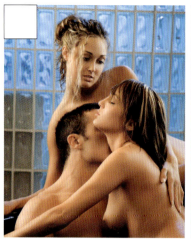

73 Ladies Locker-Room Fun

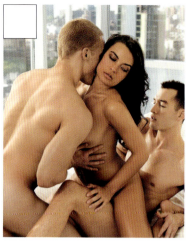

74 Oreo Cookie (and You're the Filling!)

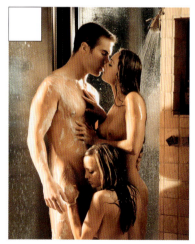

75 Merry Go Round

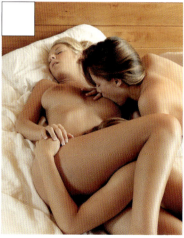

76 Three of a Kind

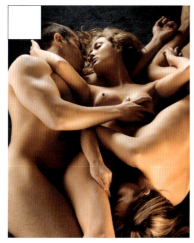

77 Daisy Chain

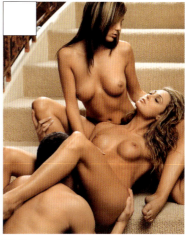

78 Queen of the Stairs

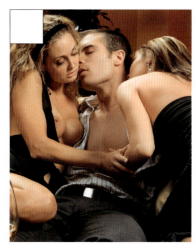

79 Twin Sisters

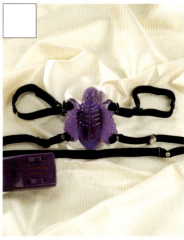

80 Remote Control

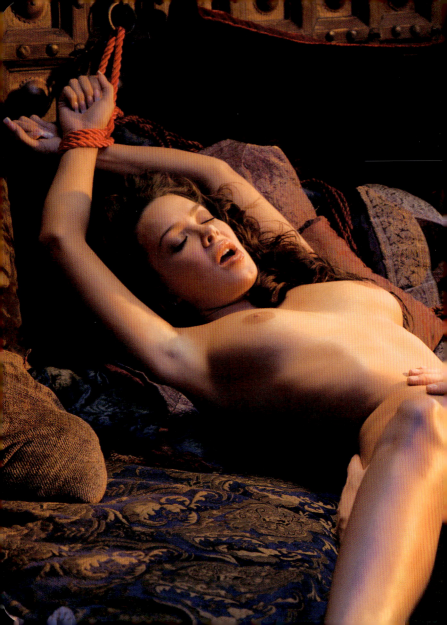

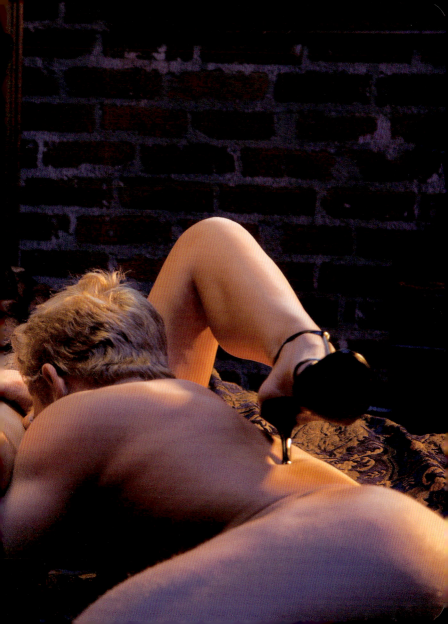

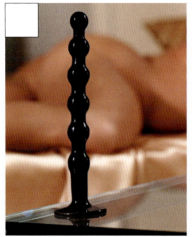

81 Pleasure Party

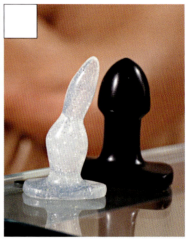

82 Backdoor Woman

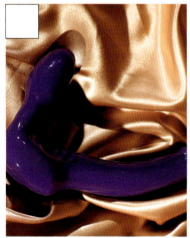

83 Good Vibrations

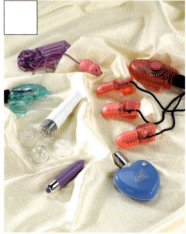

84 Finger Fun

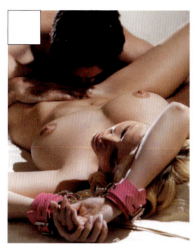

85 Tie and Tease

About the Author

Although Randi Foxx was born in the United States, she spent many years living in India. When she was eighteen, she traveled to the temples at Khajuraho, where intricate carvings illustrate explicit sexual activity. This trip led to a sexual awakening for Randi. Since then, she has dedicated her life to transforming these sacred sexual depictions into works of human art.